JUICES
& SMOOTHIES
GALORE

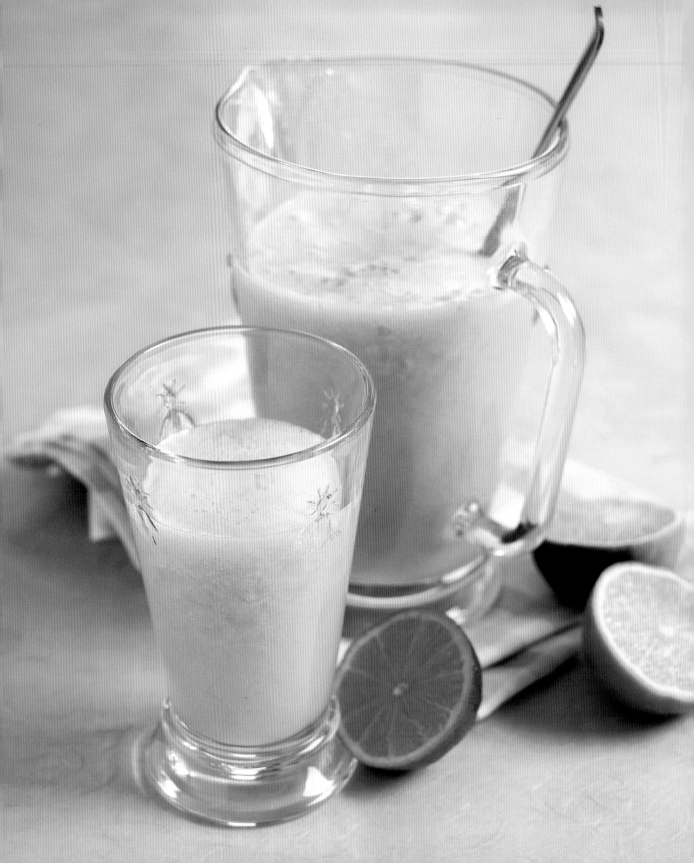

JUICES
& SMOOTHIES
GALORE

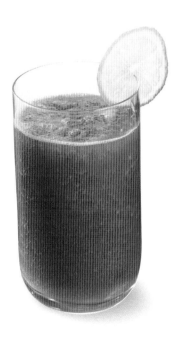

spruce

An Hachette Livre UK Company

First published in Great Britain in 2008
by Spruce, a division of
Octopus Publishing Group Ltd
2–4 Heron Quays, London E14 4JP.
www.octopusbooks.co.uk

Photography: Ian Garlick; Simon Pask
Food Styling: Eliza Baird
Page Layout: Balley Design Associates

ISBN-13: 978-1-84601-272-3

A CIP catalogue record of this book is
available from the British Library.

Printed and bound in China

10 9 8 7 6 5 4 3 2 1

This book contains the opinions and ideas of
the author. It is intended to provide helpful
and informative material on the subjects
addressed in this book and is sold with the
understanding that the author and publisher
are not engaged in rendering any kind of
personal professional services in this book.
The author and publisher disclaim all
responsibility for any liability, loss or risk,
personal or otherwise, which is incurred as
a consequence, directly or indirectly, of the
use and application of any of the contents
of this book.

CONTENTS

INTRODUCTION

When it comes to luscious liquid treats, nothing quite beats a freshly squeezed glass of juice or a super-creamy smoothie made from perfectly ripe fruit. Whether you're looking for the ultimate health kick to get your body bursting with vitality or the most indulgent glass of creamy, sweet shake you can do it with a juice or smoothie. And if you're really clever you'll manage to have a naughty treat, but get something of a health-fix at the same time by making sure it's packed with loads of healthy vitamins too!

This fabulous collection of recipes offers you something for every occasion, so you're guaranteed to find the perfect recipe no matter what your mood. Divided into seven easy-to-use chapters, you can choose from detoxifiers and power juices in The Juice Boost; invigorating veggie juices and fruity smoothies in Vital Veggies, Sweet & Fruity and Smooth & Creamy; healthy morning concoctions in Breakfast Blends; and recipes that will appeal to your more indulgent side in Frozen & Iced and Naughty But Nice. So go on — get out your juicer or blender, open your fridge and whizz yourself up a glass of something fabulous.

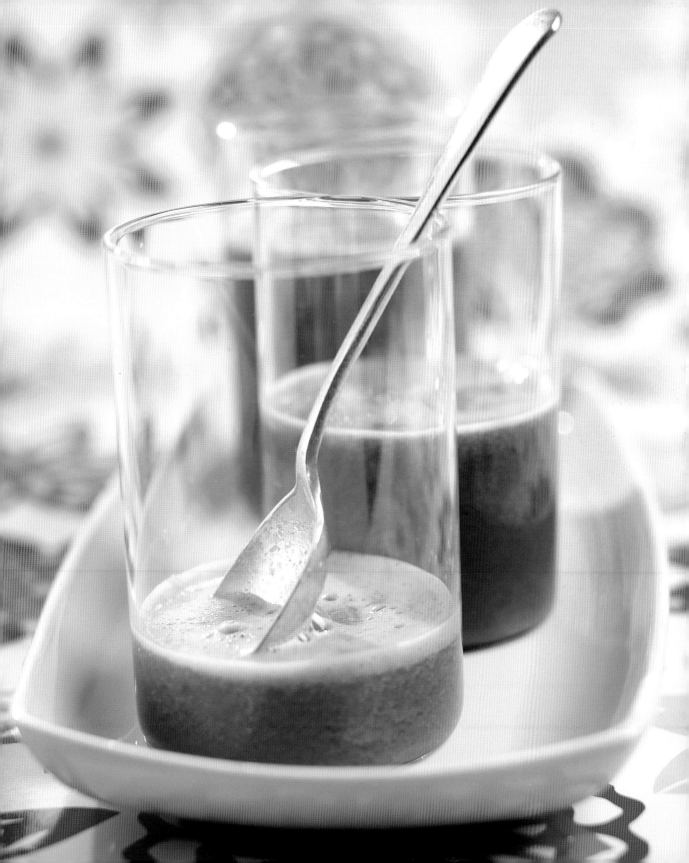

SENSATIONAL SERVING

The great thing about making your own juices and smoothies is that it means you get the absolute best out of them that you can. You control the freshness of the fruit and vegetables used, and can adjust the quantities of ingredients included to create a drink exactly to your liking. The versatility of making your own juice or smoothie is amazing.

Although shop-bought juices and smoothies might taste good, nutrients begin to deteriorate soon after juicing or blending, so to really make the most of those healthy nutrients, you need to drink the juice or smoothie as soon as you can after making it.

If you're going for a powerful health juice, pour the juice into a glass and sip it slowly. Some of the more potent vegetable juices such as wheatgrass, cabbage and beetroot can take a little getting used to – so don't gulp them down in one. Take little sips and let your body and digestion get used to the new flavours and effects.

If you're making a smoothie or juice as an indulgent treat, think about presentation. A celery or carrot stick stirrer can look stylish in a juice, while fresh berries or wedges of fruit make a stunning decoration for fruity smoothies. For more indulgent drinks, think about decorating with chocolate shavings or curls, or drizzle the glass with toffee or chocolate sauce. Try crumbling over a little meringue in a meringue smoothie or perhaps use a candy cane as a novel edible drink stirrer.

For less fussy finishes, ice is always a great addition – but whether you want to use cubes, cracked or crushed is up to you. You can also think about making colourful decorative ice cubes too. Try freezing fresh juices in ice cube trays to make coloured, flavoured ice cubes, or freeze berries, edible flowers or herbs in plain water to make ice cubes for a pretty effect.

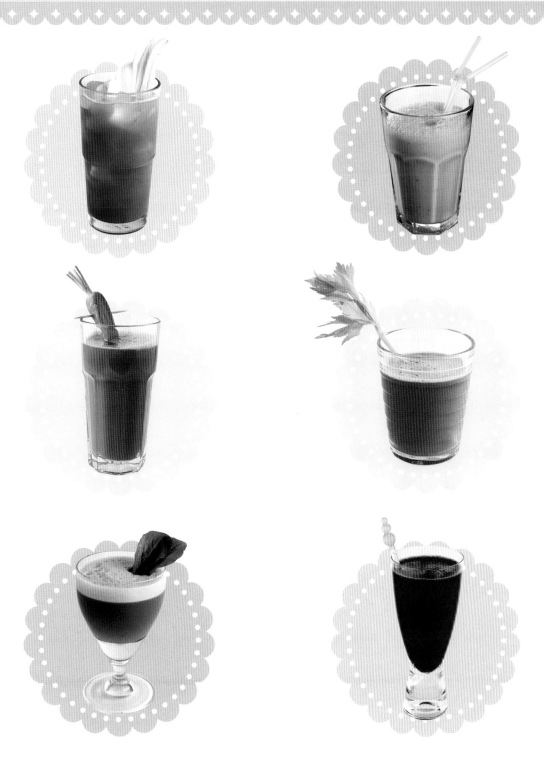

ESSENTIAL EQUIPMENT

Although juicing and blending are probably two of the simplest ways to create truly divine recipes in the kitchen you will need a couple of pieces of essential equipment to get really good results.

★ CITRUS JUICERS ★

Many electric juicers come with a cone-shaped attachment so you can juice citrus fruits quickly and easily, but there are also plenty of manual juicers that you can use to extract the juice from oranges, grapefruits, clementines, lemons and limes too. If you're only juicing a couple of fruits, the easiest and simplest juicer to use is probably a glass, ceramic or stainless steel squeezer with a ridged dome that you press the fruit down on. The best ones will have a jug underneath, or a 'moat' surrounding it, to collect the juice. They're effective but take a little more effort on the part of the person doing the juicing.

Another alternative, which is handy if you regularly juice a lot of citrus fruits, is a free-standing citrus press with a handle. You simply place the halved fruit on top of the ridged cone, then pull down the handle to force a domed 'hat' down on to the fruit to extract the juice from the fruit.

★ ELECTRIC JUICERS ★

If you want to make drinks out of vegetables and harder fruits such as apples and pears, you will need a proper electrical juicer that extracts the juice from the

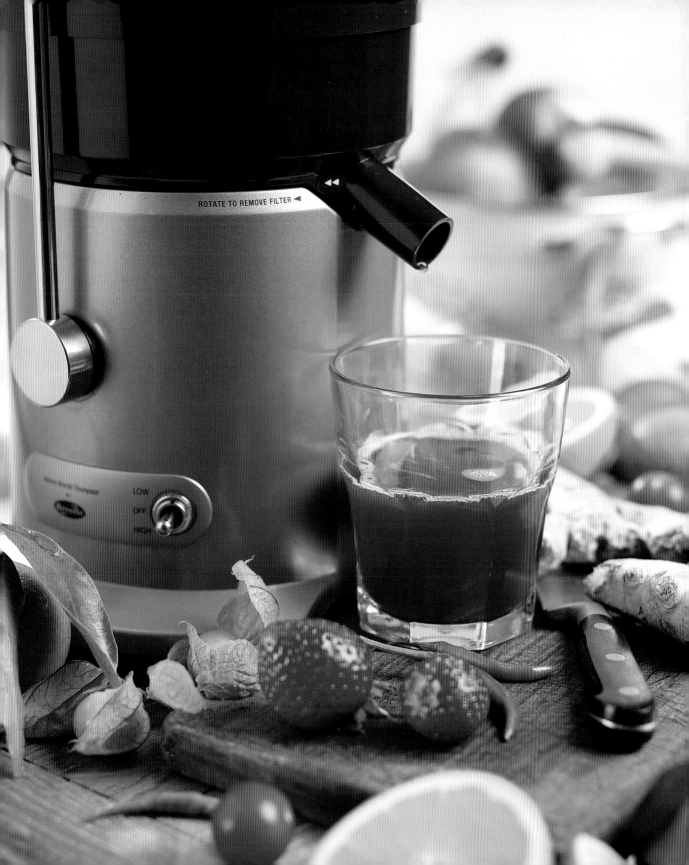

ROTATE TO REMOVE FILTER

vegetable or fruit pulp. There are two main types of juicer: centrifugal and masticating.

Centrifugal juicers finely grate the fruit and vegetable, then spin the pulp at great speed to remove the juice from the pulp by centrifugal force. These juicers tend to be more affordable and are the classic domestic juicer.

Masticating juicers are more expensive, but more efficient because they are able to extract more juice. They work by chopping the fruit and vegetables very finely to a pulp, then forcing them through a mesh to extract the juice. Different models vary in terms of efficiency and how much juice they are able to extract from the ingredients, so it's worth shopping around if you're planning on doing a lot of juicing.

★ FOOD PROCESSORS & BLENDERS ★

Essential for making smoothies, you can use any type of food processor or blender to make a smoothie.

Jug blenders are great because you can throw in all your ingredients, give it a blitz, then pour your smoothie straight into a glass with no fuss. You can even buy special 'smoothie makers', which are

essentially a jug blender with a tap at the bottom for pouring out your smoothie.

Hand-held 'wand' blenders are great for no-fuss smoothie-making because they're easy to use and wash up.

Food processors work well, but can be cumbersome when pouring out the finished smoothie, and because they're made up of several parts can be more fuss to wash up. Also keep in mind that most food processors are better suited to blending larger quantities, rather than small ones.

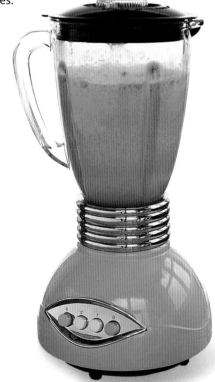

USEFUL KITCHEN BASICS

As well as the essential juicing and blending equipment, there are a few kitchen basics that are invaluable when it comes to making smoothies and juices.

★ SCRUBBING BRUSH ★

If you're using organic fruit and veg, you won't necessarily have to peel them before juicing, but you'll need to make sure that they're really well scrubbed to remove any dirt from their skins.

★ VEGETABLE PEELER ★

A good, sturdy vegetable peeler will make quick and efficient work of peeling root vegetables and hard fruits such as apples and pears. It will also be handy for removing the papery skin from fresh root ginger.

★ CHOPPING BOARD ★

You will need a good, sturdy chopping board for cutting up vegetables and fruit – either for pushing through a juicer or whizzing up in a blender. Be sure to have a separate board for chopping raw meat and fish and one for fruit and vegetables and always scrub the boards well after use.

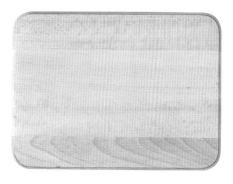

★ RUBBER SPATULA ★

These are useful for scraping down the sides of food processors and blenders during blending, and also to make sure you scrape every last drop of your finished smoothie into the glass. After all, you wouldn't want to waste any!

★ SIEVE ★

These are great for making really smooth smoothies by sieving out chunky fibres, skins or pips from fruit purées. You can also strain citrus juices through a sieve to remove the 'bits' if you prefer a smooth juice.

★ SCALES ★

The recipes in this book use quantities of fruits and vegetables – rather than weights – as much as possible, but a set of weighing scales will be useful for following some recipes.

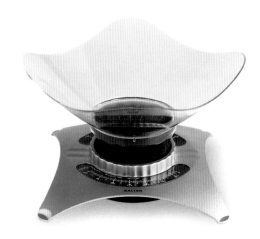

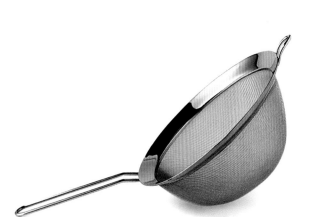

★ CHERRY PITTER ★

If you're juicing or blending cherries, you'll need to remove the stones first, and although you can do this by hand with a small knife, it's much quicker to use a special cherry pitter. You simply fit the cherry into the cup of the cherry pitter and then squeeze the handles together to draw a bar through the cherry and eject the stone through the other side.

★ KNIVES ★

Make sure you have a couple of good, sharp knives, including a large, heavy one that can deal with chopping up large fruits such as melons and pineapples.

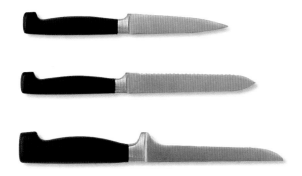

★ MEASURING JUG, CUPS & SPOONS ★

You'll need these to accurately measure volumes of liquid such as milk, juice, yogurt and honey as well as dry ingredients such as spices and sugar.

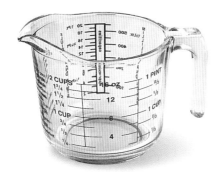

★ ICE CREAM SCOOP ★

A sturdy ice cream scoop is ideal for scooping up perfect balls of ice cream or sorbet to drop into smoothies or shakes. They're designed to deal with hard ices so you don't have to risk bending your spoons. There are loads of different scoops on the market, from the simplest scoops on a thick handle to ones with levers to help release the ball of ice cream.

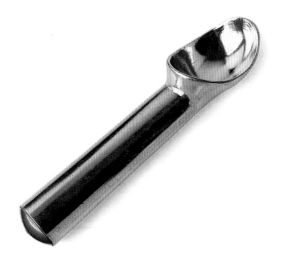

INGREDIENTS

As with all cooking, the better your ingredients, the better the end result will be when you're juicing and blending. A really well-flavoured carrot or tomato will make a truly fabulous, mouthwatering juice, while watery specimens will produce weaker, less well-flavoured juices.

★ FRUIT & VEG FOR JUICING ★

You can pretty much juice any fruit, vegetable or leaf except bananas, which just don't give out juice. Choose well-flavoured specimens in peak condition. Don't be tempted to use over-ripe fruit. Juicing seems to intensify the sweetness of fruits and vegetables, and using very ripe fruits, which are naturally very sweet, will produce very sweet juices.

★ FRUITS FOR BLENDING ★

Soft fruits such as berries, stone fruits and soft tropical fruits are perfect for blending because they whizz up to smooth, juicy purées without becoming too pulpy. Harder fruits such as apples and pears are better for juicing because they become too thick and fibrous when blended rather than smooth and creamy. However, this doesn't mean you can't add these ingredients to your smoothies – simply juice them first, then add to the soft fruits in the blender and blend until smooth.

★ CREAMY SMOOTHIES ★

Dairy products are a popular addition to smoothies – whether it's a splash of milk, a spoonful of yogurt or custard, a drizzle of cream or a scoop of ice cream. However, if you want a creamy smoothie but want to keep it dairy-free, there are all kinds of other ingredients you can use instead. Dairy-free milks, such as soya, oat, nut and rice milks, are great for smoothies and add their own distinct flavour. Silken tofu blends

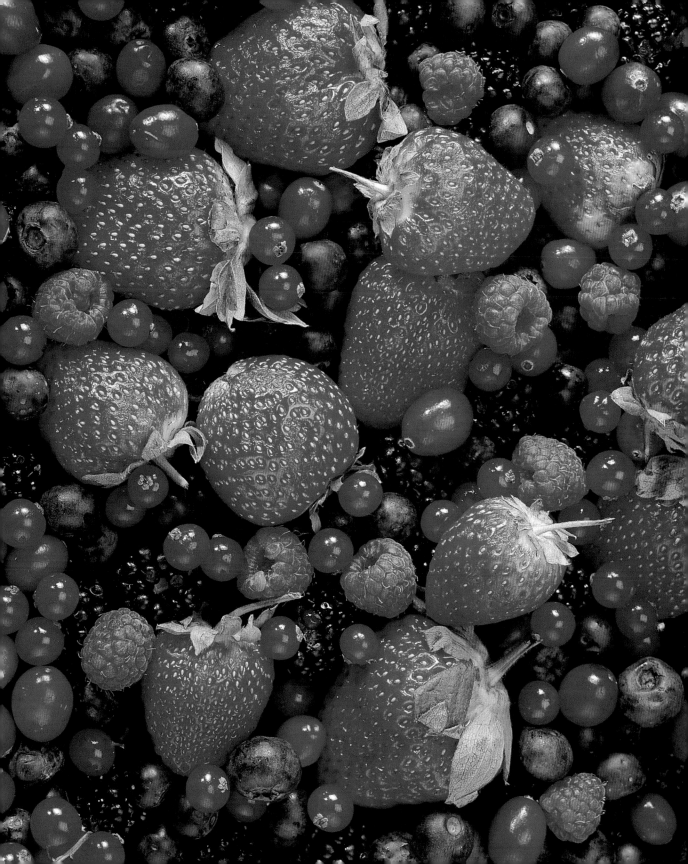

up to a silky, smooth, creamy consistency that's just divine when combined with soft, ripe fruits, while creamy soya desserts offer a good alternative to yogurt.

★ KEEPING IT SWEET ★

As well as the natural sweetness provided by ripe fruits and vegetables, you may want to add other sweeteners to juices and smoothies. Honey is a popular choice as the natural sugars in honey are kinder to the body than refined sugars and complement the other healthy ingredients in many juices and smoothies. However, there are plenty of other sweeteners too, including white and brown sugars, molasses with its intense flavour, dulce de leche (toffee syrup) and chocolate syrup – both of which add sweetness and flavour.

★ OTHER FLAVOURINGS & ADDITIONS ★

Once you've got the basics of fruits, vegetables, dairy products and sweeteners, you can start adding other ingredients to your smoothies. Simple flavourings such as coffee, chocolate (melted or cocoa powder) and vanilla are always popular choices, but you can also be adventurous too. Try adding brownies, meringues or nougat, or adding a splash of spirit or liqueur such as Grand Marnier or brandy. Sorbet, ice cream and frozen yogurt are great in iced smoothies and shakes, while chocolate shavings and curls can be great for decorations. For added flavour, ingredients such as lemon and orange curd can add both sweetness and zest, while nuts, muesli and dried fruit can add both body, texture and taste.

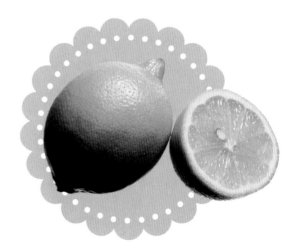

PERFECT JUICING & BLENDING

There isn't much of a secret to juicing and blending. As long as you're using great-tasting ingredients, including produce that is both ripe and fresh, it's pretty hard to go wrong. There are, however, a few rules of thumb that will help you achieve great results every time.

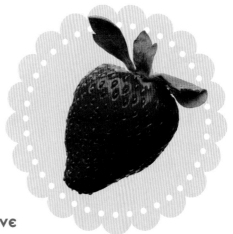

1. ALWAYS WASH UP YOUR JUICER AS SOON AS YOU'VE USED IT

No matter how much you spend on your juicer, there's no getting away from the fact that they're a bit of a pain to wash up. There are generally several pieces to take apart and each bit will need a good scrub. When you do it straight away, it will take mere minutes, however, if you decide to leave your juicer to dry with bits of pulp and juice attached – the task of washing up will be a gargantuan one.

2. WHAT ORDER TO JUICE?

As a general rule, put smaller or less juicy items such as ginger, chilli or spinach through the juicer first, then 'flush' the juice through with larger, juicier items such as carrots or apples.

3. DEALING WITH STRONG FLAVOURS

Some ingredients can have very strong, overpowering flavours so you only need to use a little bit and 'dilute' it with a milder base juice. For example, cabbage and celery both have quite strong flavours, so a little goes a long way. If you find you've put too much of a strong ingredient in your juice, add more of your milder-flavoured ingredients such as carrots or apples.

4. ENHANCING FLAVOURS

If your smoothie or juice tastes a little bland, often all it needs is a good squeeze of lemon or lime juice to pep up the flavours and enhance the tastes that are already there. For example, mango has an intense, fragrant, sweet flavour but is vastly improved by a good squeeze of lime juice, which can transform a sweet, fruity smoothie into something utterly tantalizing and tongue-tingling.

5. THINNING SMOOTHIES

Some fruits will create smoothies that are more of a purée than a drink and are just too thick to sip so you'll need to dilute them. A splash of milk or a complementary fruit juice are usually good choices. If the smoothie is very sweet and strongly flavoured, you may simply be able to add a splash of water.

6. THICKENING SMOOTHIES

If your smoothie is too thin, try adding a spoonful of yogurt, créme fraîche or thick cream to give it more body. Alternatively, add a small quantity of banana, mango or avocado, all of which will help to thicken it.

7. SMOOTHING OUT SMOOTHIES

Some ingredients such as pineapple can be quite fibrous and can make rather pulpy smoothies, so you may want to remove some of the fibres after blending. Simply pour the smoothie into a sieve and press through using the back of a spoon.

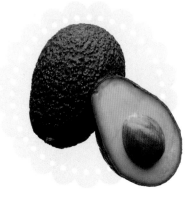

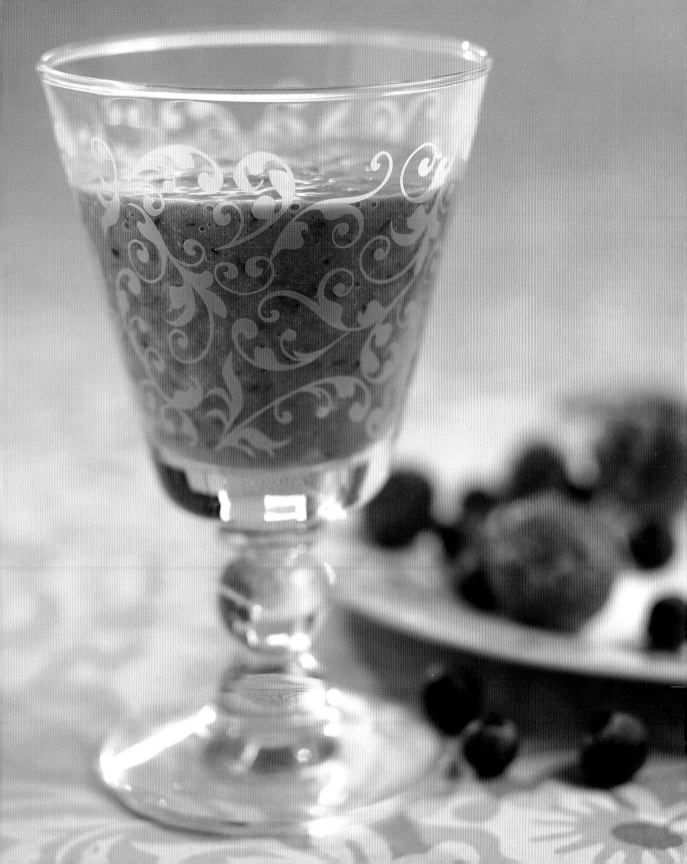

VEGETABLE	ENERGY (Kj)	ENERGY (kCAL)	PROTEIN (g)	FIBRE (total dietary)	CALCIUM (mg)	PHOSPHO-RUS (mg)	IRON (mg)	POTASSIUM (mg)	MAGNESIUM (mg)
artichoke, globe	197	47	3.27	5.4	44	90	1.28	370	60
asparagus	96	23	2.28	2.1	21	56	0.87	273	18
avocado	674	161	1.98	5	11	41	1.02	599	39
beans, green	130	31	1.82	3.4	37	38	1.04	209	25
beetroot	180	43	1.61	2.8	16	40	0.8	325	23
broccoli	117	28	2.98	3	48	66	0.88	325	25
cabbage	105	25	1.44	2.3	47	23	0.59	246	15
carrot	180	43	1.03	3	27	44	0.5	323	15
cauliflower	105	25	1.98	2.5	22	44	0.44	303	15
celeriac	176	42	1.5	1.8	43	115	0.7	300	20
celery	67	16	0.75	1.7	40	25	0.4	287	11
cucumber	54	13	0.69	0.8	14	20	0.26	144	11
fennel, bulb	130	31	1.24	3.1	49	50	0.73	414	17
lettuce, cos or romaine	59	14	1.62	1.7	36	45	1.1	290	6
lettuce, iceberg	50	12	1.01	1.4	19	20	0.5	158	9
parsnips	314	75	1.2	4.9	36	71	0.59	375	29
peas	339	42	2.8	2.6	43	53	2.08	200	24
peppers, green	113	27	0.89	1.8	9	19	0.46	177	10
peppers, red	113	27	0.89	2	9	19	0.46	177	10
peppers, yellow	113	27	1	0.9	11	24	0.46	212	12
potatoes	331	79	2.07	1.6	7	46	0.76	543	21
radish	84	20	0.6	1.6	21	18	0.29	232	9
rocket	105	25	2.58	1.6	160	52	1.46	369	47
spinach	92	22	2.86	2.7	99	49	2.71	558	79
squash	84	20	1.18	1.9	20	35	0.46	195	23
tomatoes	88	21	0.85	1.1	5	24	0.45	222	11
watercress	46	11	2.3	1.5	120	60	0.2	330	21

value given is per 100g of edible portion   * indicates data is not available   Source: US Department of Agricultural Research Service

ZINC (mg)	MANGANESE (mg)	SELENIUM (mcg)	VITAMIN A (iu)	VITAMIN E (mg)	THIAMIN (mg)	RIBOFLAVIN (mg)	NIACIN (mg)	VITAMIN B6 (mg)	VITAMIN C (mg)
0.49	0.26	0.2	185	0.19	0.07	0.07	1.05	0.12	11.7
0.46	0.26	2.3	583	2	0.14	0.13	1.17	0.13	13.2
0.42	0.23	0.4	612	1.34	0.11	0.12	1.92	0.28	7.9
0.24	0.21	0.6	668	0.41	0.08	0.11	0.75	0.07	16.3
0.35	0.33	0.7	38	0.3	0.03	0.04	0.33	0.07	4.9
0.4	0.23	3	1542	1.66	0.07	0.12	0.64	0.16	93.2
0.18	0.16	0.9	133	0.11	0.05	0.04	0.3	0.1	32.2
0.2	0.14	1.1	28129	0.46	0.1	0.06	0.93	0.15	9.3
0.28	0.16	0.6	19	0.04	0.06	0.06	0.53	0.22	46.4
0.33	0.16	0.7	0	0.36	0.05	0.06	0.7	0.17	8
0.13	0.1	0.9	134	0.36	0.05	0.05	0.32	0.09	7
0.2	0.08	0	215	0.08	0.02	0.02	0.22	0.04	5.3
0.2	0.19	0.7	134	*	0.01	0.03	0.64	0.05	12
0.25	0.64	0.2	2600	0.44	0.1	0.1	0.5	0.05	24
0.22	0.15	0.2	330	0.28	0.05	0.03	0.19	0.04	3.9
0.59	0.56	1.8	0	*	0.09	0.05	0.7	0.09	17
0.27	0.24	0.7	145	0.39	0.15	0.08	0.6	0.16	60
0.12	0.12	0.3	632	0.69	0.07	0.03	0.51	0.25	89.3
0.12	0.12	0.3	5700	0.69	0.07	0.03	0.51	0.25	190
0.17	0.12	0.3	238	*	0.03	0.03	0.89	0.17	183.5
0.39	0.26	0.3	0	0.06	0.09	0.04	1.48	0.26	19.7
0.3	0.07	0.7	8	0	0.01	0.05	0.3	0.07	22.8
0.47	0.32	0.3	2373	0.43	0.04	0.09	0.31	0.07	15
0.53	0.9	1	6715	1.89	0.08	0.19	0.72	0.2	28.1
0.26	0.16	0.2	196	0.12	0.06	0.04	0.55	0.11	14.8
0.09	0.11	0.4	623	0.38	0.06	0.05	0.63	0.08	10
0.11	0.24	0.9	4700	1	0.09	0.12	0.2	0.13	43

FRUIT	ENERGY (Kj)	ENERGY (kCAL)	PROTEIN (g)	FIBRE (total dietary)	VITAMIN A (iu)	THIAMIN vitamin B1 (mg)	RIBOFLAVIN vitamin B2 (mg)	NIACIN vitamin B3 (mg)	VITAMIN B6 (mg)
apple	247	59	0.19	2.7	53	0.02	0.01	0.08	0.05
apricot	201	48	1.4	2.4	2612	0.03	0.04	0.6	0.05
banana	385	92	1.03	2.4	81	0.05	0.1	0.54	0.58
blackberry	218	52	0.72	5.3	165	0.03	0.04	0.4	0.06
blueberry	234	56	0.67	2.7	100	0.05	0.05	0.36	0.04
cherry, glacé	301	72	1.2	2.3	214	0.05	0.06	0.4	0.04
cherry, sour	209	50	1	1.6	1283	0.03	0.04	0.4	0.04
cranberry	205	49	0.39	4.2	46	0.03	0.02	0.1	0.07
date	1151	275	1.97	7.5	50	0.09	0.1	2.2	0.19
fig	310	74	0.75	3.3	142	0.06	0.05	0.4	0.11
grapefruit, pink and red	126	30	0.55	*	259	0.03	0.02	0.19	0.04
grapes, red or white	297	71	0.66	1	73	0.09	0.06	0.3	0.11
kiwi	255	61	0.99	3.4	175	0.02	0.05	0.5	0.09
lemon	84	20	1.2	4.7	30	0.05	0.04	0.2	0.11
lime	126	30	0.7	2.8	10	0.03	0.02	0.2	0.04
mango	272	65	0.51	1.8	3894	0.06	0.06	0.58	0.13
melon, cantaloupe	146	35	0.88	0.8	3224	0.04	0.02	0.57	0.12
melon, honeydew	146	35	0.46	0.6	40	0.08	0.02	0.6	0.06
nectarine	205	49	0.94	1.6	736	0.02	0.04	0.99	0.03
orange	197	47	0.94	2.4	205	0.09	0.04	0.28	0.06
papaya	163	39	0.61	1.8	284	0.03	0.03	0.34	0.02
passion fruit	406	97	2.2	10.4	700	0	0.13	1.5	0.1
peach	180	43	0.7	2	535	0.02	0.04	0.99	0.02
pear	59	59	0.39	2.4	20	0.02	0.04	0.1	0.02
physallis	222	53	1.9	*	720	0.11	0.04	2.8	*
pineapple	205	49	0.39	1.2	23	0.09	0.04	0.42	0.09
plum	230	55	0.79	1.5	323	0.04	0.1	0.5	0.08
pomegranate	285	68	0.95	0.6	0	0.03	0.03	0.3	0.11
raspberry	205	49	0.91	6.8	130	0.03	0.09	0.9	0.06
rhubarb	88	21	0.9	1.8	100	0.02	0.03	0.3	0.02
sharon fruit	531	127	*	*	*	*	*	*	*
strawberry	126	30	0.61	2.3	27	0.02	0.07	0.23	0.06

value given is per 100g of edible portion   * indicates data is not available   Source: US Department of Agricultural Research Service

VITAMIN E (mg)	CALCIUM (mg)	PHOSPHORUS (mg)	IRON (mg)	POTASSIUM (mg)	MAGNESIUM (mg)	ZINC (mg)	MANGANESE (mcg)	SELENIUM (mcg)	VITAMIN C (mg)
0.32	7	7	0.18	115	5	0.04	0.05	0.3	5.7
0.89	14	19	0.54	296	8	0.26	0.08	0.4	10
0.27	6	20	0.31	396	29	0.16	0.15	1.1	9.1
0.71	32	21	0.57	196	20	0.27	1.29	0.6	21
1	6	10	0.17	89	5	0.11	0.28	0.6	13
0.13	15	19	0.39	224	11	0.06	0.09	0.6	7
0.13	16	15	0.32	179	9	0.1	0.11	0.4	10
0.1	7	9	0.2	71	5	0.13	0.16	0.6	13.5
0.1	32	40	0.15	652	35	0.29	0.3	1.9	*
0.89	35	14	0.37	232	17	0.15	0.13	0.6	2
*	11	9	0.12	129	8	0.07	0.01	*	38.1
0.7	11	13	0.26	185	6	0.05	0.06	0.2	10.8
1.12	26	40	0.41	332	30	0.17	*	0.6	98
*	61	15	0.7	145	12	0.1	*	*	77
0.24	33	18	0.6	102	6	0.11	0.01	0.4	29.1
1.12	10	11	0.13	156	9	0.04	0.03	0.6	27.7
0.15	11	17	0.21	309	11	0.16	0.05	0.4	42.2
0.15	6	10	0.07	271	7	0.07	0.02	0.4	24.8
0.89	5	16	0.15	212	8	0.09	0.04	0.4	5.4
0.24	40	14	0.1	181	10	0.07	0.03	0.5	53.2
1.12	24	5	0.1	257	10	0.07	0.01	0.6	61.8
1.12	12	68	1.6	348	29	0.1	*	0.6	30
0.7	5	12	0.11	197	7	0.14	0.05	0.4	6.6
0.5	11	11	0.25	125	6	0.12	0.08	1	4
*	9	40	1	*	*	*	*	*	*
0.1	7	7	0.37	113	14	0.08	1.65	0.6	15.4
0.6	4	10	0.1	172	7	0.1	0.05	0.5	9.5
0.55	3	8	0.3	259	3	0.12	*	0.6	6.1
0.45	22	12	0.57	152	18	0.46	1.01	0.6	25
0.2	86	14	0.22	288	12	0.1	0.2	1.1	8
*	27	26	2.5	310	*	*	*	*	66
0.14	14	19	0.38	166	10	0.13	0.29	0.7	56.7

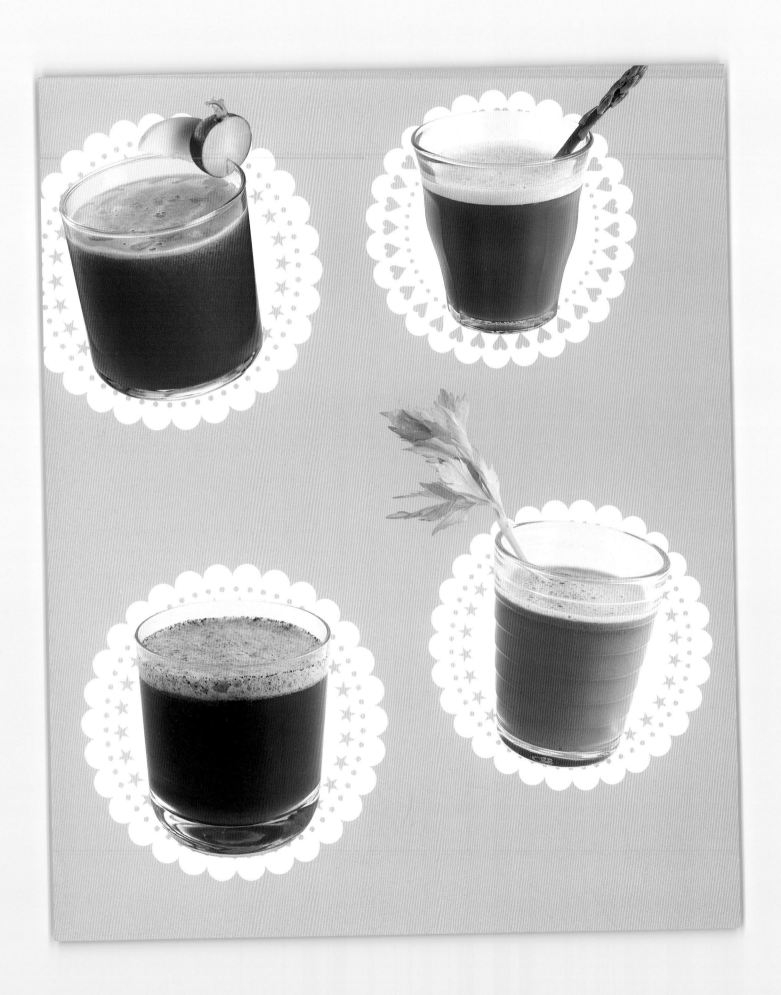

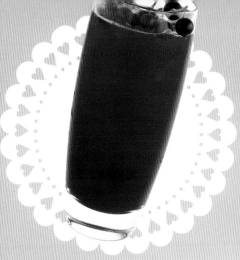
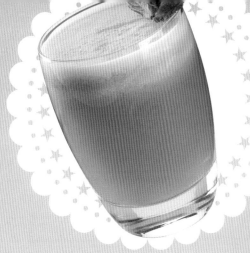

THE JUICE BOOST

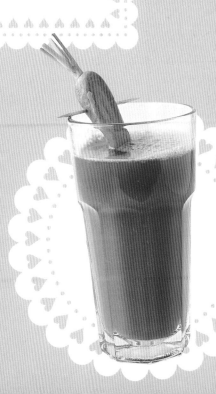
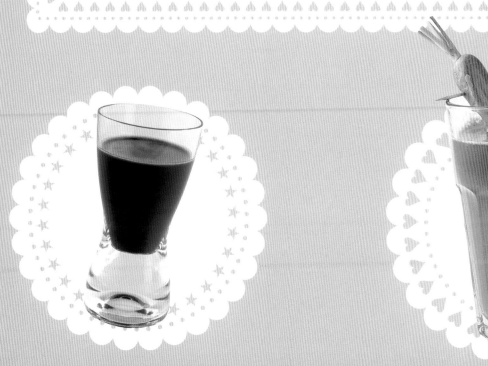

THE BIG BEETROOT BOOSTER

GINGER, BEETROOT & ORANGE

This sweet, intensely flavoured juice with the peppery bite of ginger is jam-packed with vitamins and nutrients that are guaranteed to get your whole system firing on all cylinders. If you want it for pure booster value, serve it as it is, but for a refresher, add a splash of water and serve over ice.

MAKES 1 GLASS

1cm piece of fresh root ginger
2 fresh beetroot, roughly chopped
2 oranges, halved

1. Press the ginger and beetroot through a juicer.

2. Squeeze the juice from the oranges and stir it into the beetroot and ginger juice. Pour into a glass and serve immediately.

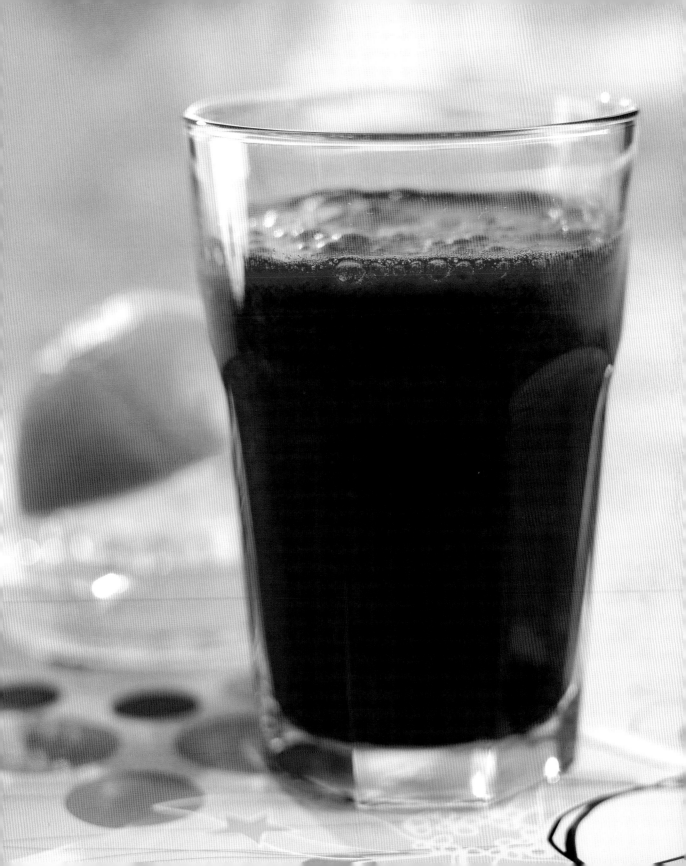

TOXIN BUSTER

APPLE, CARROT, TOMATO, CELERY & MILK THISTLE

Every ingredient in this cleansing juice helps to stimulate the liver and remove toxins from the body. Milk thistle, which is available from health-food stores, is an important liver-supporting herb. Tomatoes, carrots and celery stimulate the liver, and apples help to remove toxins from it.

MAKES 1 GLASS

½ apple
2 carrots, trimmed
100g cherry tomatoes
2 celery sticks, plus an extra stick,
   to decorate
¼ teaspoon milk thistle extract

1. Roughly chop the apple and carrots. Press the tomatoes through a juicer, followed by the apple, carrots and celery.

2. Stir the milk thistle extract into the juice, then pour into a glass and add a leafy celery stick as a healthy, liver-stimulating stirrer.

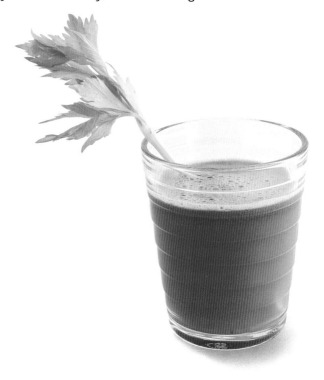

POPEYE'S FINEST

SPINACH, APPLE & SPIRULINA

Adding spirulina to this vibrant green juice transforms it from a healthy cleanser into a turbo-charged power-purifier. Combining iron-rich spinach with vitamin C-rich apples helps to ensure the maximum absorption of nutrients, and also makes a deliciously mild, fruity blend.

MAKES 1 GLASS

120g baby spinach, plus extra
    to decorate (optional)
3 small dessert apples
1/4 teaspoon spirulina

1. Wash the spinach and drain well, then roughly chop the apples. Press the spinach through a juicer, alternating with chunks of apple.

2. Stir the spirulina into the juice and pour into a glass. Decorate with a few baby spinach leaves, if liked, and serve immediately.

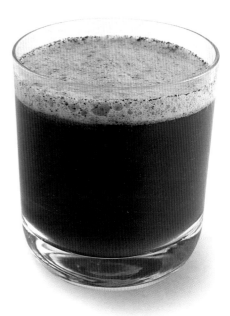

GREEN GIANT

SUGAR SNAP PEAS, ASPARAGUS & FENNEL

Fennel helps to flush toxins out of the system, while
calming the stomach at the same time. Paired with sweet,
stimulating sugar snap peas and kidney-boosting asparagus,
it makes a deliciously refreshing, aniseed-flavoured juice.

MAKES 1 GLASS

120g sugar snap peas
3 asparagus spears, plus 1 spear
   to decorate
1 fennel bulb, roughly chopped

1. Push the sugar snaps through the juicer, followed by the asparagus and
chunks of fennel.
2. Stir the juice and pour into a glass. Decorate with an asparagus spear
and serve immediately.

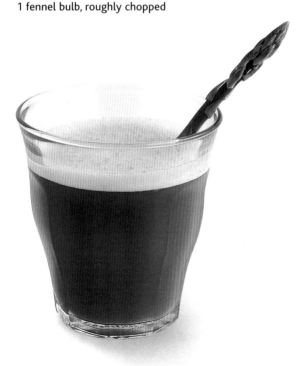

MINTY PINEAPPLE PUNCH

PEPPERMINT, PINEAPPLE & ORANGE

This tall, refreshing juice is a great thirst quencher and is simply bursting with immune-boosting vitamin C. Calming peppermint tea aids the digestive system, along with zingy pineapple, and also adds a certain something to the flavour that's quite irresistible.

MAKES 1 GLASS

1 peppermint tea bag
250ml boiling water
275g peeled pineapple (about 8cm),
    roughly chopped
2 oranges, halved
Fresh mint leaves, to decorate

1. Put the peppermint tea bag in a jug, pour over the boiling water and steep for 5 minutes. Remove the tea bag and leave to cool completely.
2. Press the pineapple through a juicer. Squeeze the juice from the oranges and stir into the pineapple juice with 125ml of the cooled mint tea. Pour into a glass, decorate with fresh mint leaves and serve immediately.

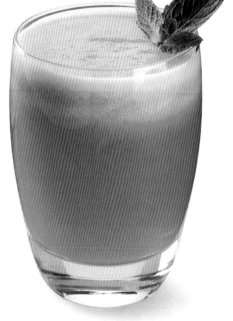

MELLOW YELLOW

MANGO, MELON, TURMERIC & LEMON

In natural medicine, mangoes are said to purify the blood, whereas fleshy melons are a great diuretic and help to cleanse the kidneys. Turmeric is a perfect partner to their sweet, aromatic juice and helps the body release toxins.

MAKES 1 GLASS

1 mango
¼ large cantaloupe melon
   (about 450g)
¼ teaspoon turmeric
2 teaspoons lemon juice

1. Using a small, sharp knife, remove the peel from the mango, then slice the flesh away from the stone.

2. Scoop out and discard the seeds from the melon, and then cut the fruit into slices. Remove the skin and cut the flesh into large chunks.

3. Press the mango through a juicer, followed by the melon, then stir in the turmeric and lemon juice. Pour into a glass and serve immediately.

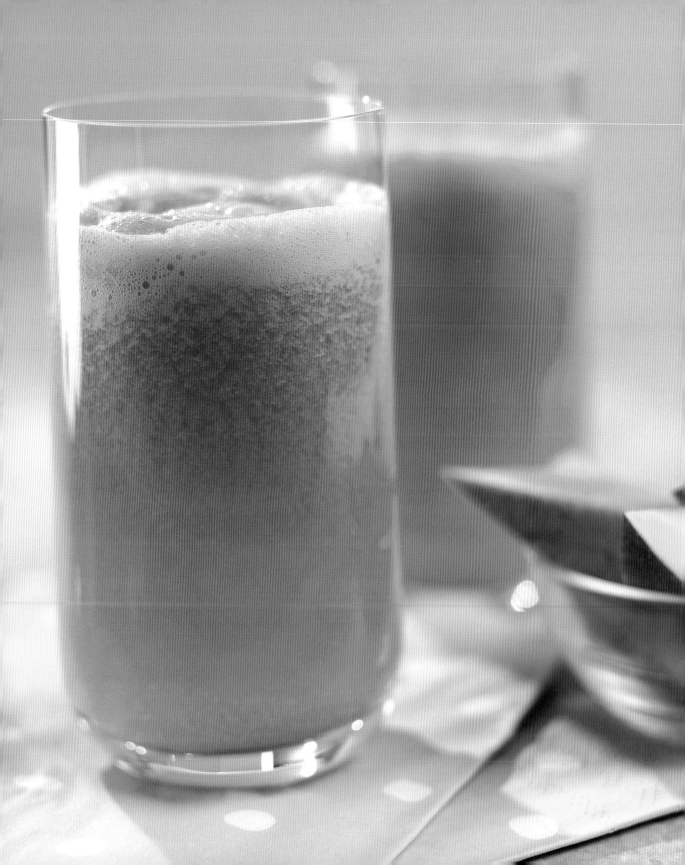

CLEANSING POWERS

WHEATGRASS

A shot of this juice and your body won't know what's hit it. Renowned for its detoxifying properties, wheatgrass is the king of cleansers. It's powerful stuff though, so sip this juice slowly as some people can feel slightly nauseous and light-headed the first time they try it. You need an awful lot of wheatgrass to make a small glass, but the benefits are worth the effort!

MAKES 1 SHOT

80g wheatgrass

1. Push small handfuls of the wheatgrass through a juicer. (Juicing wheatgrass is a tough job so you'll need a powerful juicer. Don't try to juice too much grass at once, as it can get caught up in some machines.)
2. Pour the juice into a shot glass and drink straight away, taking tiny sips.

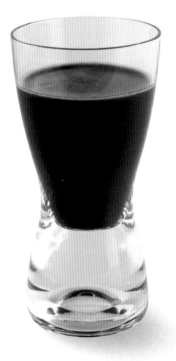

GROWING YOUR OWN WHEATGRASS

You can often buy trays of wheatgrass from health-food and organic shops, but it is easy to grow your own at home. Place 250g whole wheat grains in a bowl, pour over cold water and leave to soak for 24 hours. Fill a tray (measuring about 30 x 40cm) with about 4cm organic compost and spray lightly with water. Drain the wheat grains and scatter them over the compost, pressing them in slightly. Leave in a warm, sunny place. Check every day and spray with water (being careful not to over-water). In less than a week, you should have a tray full of wheatgrass ready for juicing.

HELL'S FIRE

CHILLI, BUTTERNUT SQUASH & PEAR

This intensely sweet, fiery hot juice is guaranteed to blow
out the cobwebs. Try to find Thai chillies – their intense,
ferocious heat contrasts wonderfully with the thick, syrupy
butternut squash juice.

MAKES 1 SMALL GLASS

1 small green chilli
240g butternut squash
³/₄ pear

1. Remove the seeds and white pith from the chilli, mince finely and set aside.

2. Peel the squash and roughly chop the flesh. Roughly chop the pear.

3. Press the squash and pear through a juicer and then whisk in the chilli. Pour into a small glass and serve immediately.

CARROT & CELERY SURPRISE!

CARROT, CELERY & GRAPE

This vibrant veggie juice is so sweet, you'd almost never guess it was made with a vegetable also, so it makes the perfect choice if you're new to juicing. Packed with vitamins and nutrients, it'll act as a real pick-me-up when you're feeling low.

MAKES 1 GLASS

4 carrots, trimmed
1 celery stick, plus an extra stick to decorate
175g white grapes

1. Roughly chop the carrots, then press through a juicer with the celery and grapes.
2. Pour the juice into a glass, decorate with a celery stick stirrer and serve immediately.

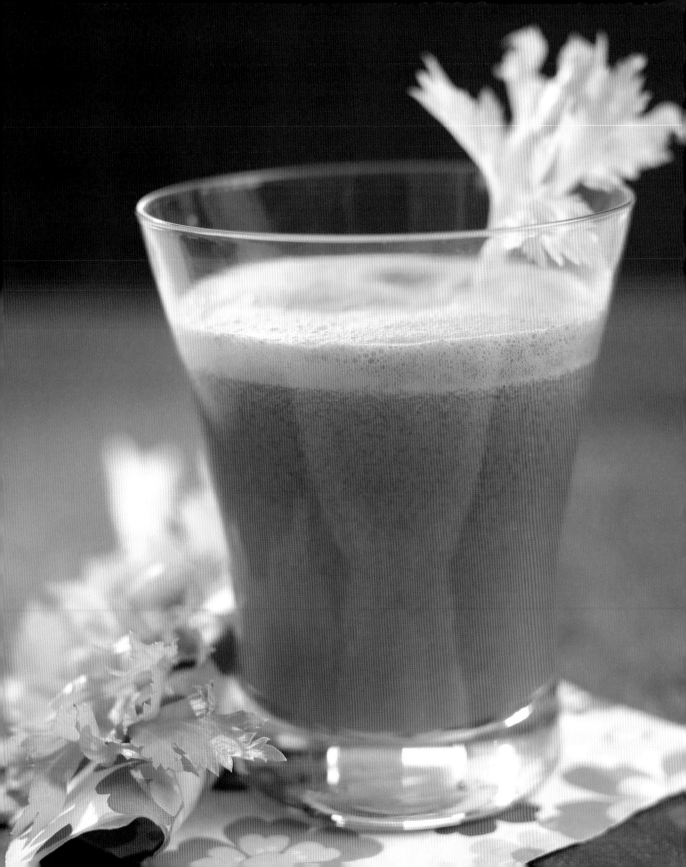

DETOX-IFICATION

GINGER, CARROT, APPLE & PEAR

Carrots, apples and pears are packed with nutrients and have the added bonus of being great detoxifiers. Drink a large glass of this sweet, mild juice and feel its cleansing action start to work almost immediately. Pears are said to ensure a clear complexion and glossy hair too so you'll notice the benefits in no time.

MAKES 1 TALL GLASS

2cm piece of fresh root ginger
3 large carrots
1 sharp-tasting dessert apple
1 pear
1 baby carrot with green leaves, to
  decorate (optional)

JUICE TIP
Carrots and apples make a great base for loads of juices and go well with both fruits and vegetables. Try ringing the changes by adding beetroot, orange or tomato in place of the pear and ginger – or if you're feeling daring, try a combination of all three!

1. Thinly peel the ginger, then scrub the carrots well and remove both ends. Wash the apple and pear, and cut the carrots and fruit into large chunks.

2. Press the ginger through a juicer, followed by the carrots, apple and pear. Stir the mixture to ensure all the juices are combined, and then pour into a tall glass. Decorate with a baby carrot stirrer, if liked, and serve immediately.

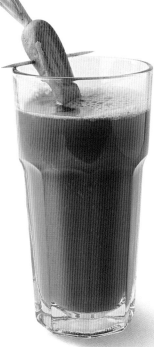

GREEN ICE

WATERCRESS & CELERY

Not to everybody's taste, this strong, bitter, peppery juice can take a little getting used to. But the benefits really do outweigh the tingling effect it has on the taste buds. Celery cleanses and supports the liver, and helps flush out toxins at the same time. Watercress is packed with magnesium, calcium and iron, and also contains sulphur, which helps to rejuvenate the hair and nails.

MAKES 1 GLASS

20g watercress
5 celery sticks
Ice cubes, to serve (optional)

1. Press the watercress through a juicer, followed by the celery sticks.

2. Pour the juice into a glass and add a few ice cubes, if liked. Sip slowly, or gulp down as quickly as you can.

RAVISHING RADISH JUICE

RADISH, TOMATO & APPLE

This lovely pinky orange juice has a really fresh, slightly peppery taste from the radishes and a natural astringency that makes it taste as though it's doing you the power of good. The tomatoes and apples are choc-full of vitamins and nutrients to fire up your body, while the pectin in the apples will help to cleanse your system.

MAKES **1 SMALL GLASS**

Large handful of radishes, halved
2 ripe tomatoes, roughly chopped
1 apple, roughly chopped

1. Push the radishes, tomatoes and apple through a juicer setting aside 1 radish half and a slice of apple to decorate, if liked.

2. Give the juice a stir, then pour into a small glass, decorate with the radish and apple, if using, and serve immediately.

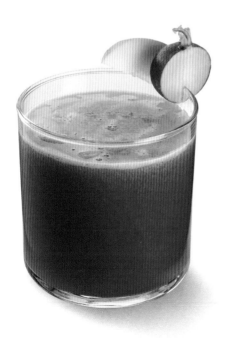

PURPLE RAIN

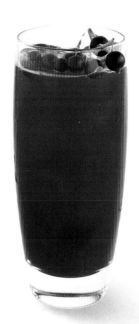

BEETROOT, APPLE & BLACKCURRANT

Packed with immune-boosting vitamin C, beta-carotene and body-building iron, this sweet, fruity juice is guaranteed to kick-start your whole system and keep it running at peak performance. Using cooked beetroot gives an intensely sweet juice, but you can use raw for a more potent taste if preferred.

MAKES 1 TALL GLASS

2 cooked beetroots
1 apple
60g blackcurrants, plus extra
   to decorate
2 tablespoons water
Ice cubes, to serve

1. Roughly chop the beetroots and apple. Press the blackcurrants through a juicer followed by the chunks of beetroot and apple.

2. Stir in the cold water to dilute the juice, pour into a tall glass filled with ice cubes and serve decorated with blackcurrants.

JUICE TIP
When blackcurrants are out of season, you can use frozen berries instead. Leave them to thaw, then press through the juicer as you would fresh currants.

WATERMELON & APPLE REFRESHER

STAR ANISE, WATERMELON & APPLE

This light, refreshing juice is great for keeping you hydrated. Watermelon is rich in cancer-fighting lycopene, while apples are a great detox fruit. Choose sharp, well-flavoured apples such as Cox's or Braeburns to offset the mild sweetness of the watermelon.

MAKES 1 GLASS

125ml water
1 star anise
1 slice (about 275g) of watermelon
1½ apples, roughly chopped

1. Put the star anise in a small pan with the water. Bring to the boil, reduce the heat and simmer for 5 minutes. Remove from the heat and leave to cool for 30 minutes.

2. Remove the skin from the watermelon and roughly chop the flesh, then press through a juicer with the apples. Stir the star anise-flavoured water into the juice, then pour into a glass and serve.

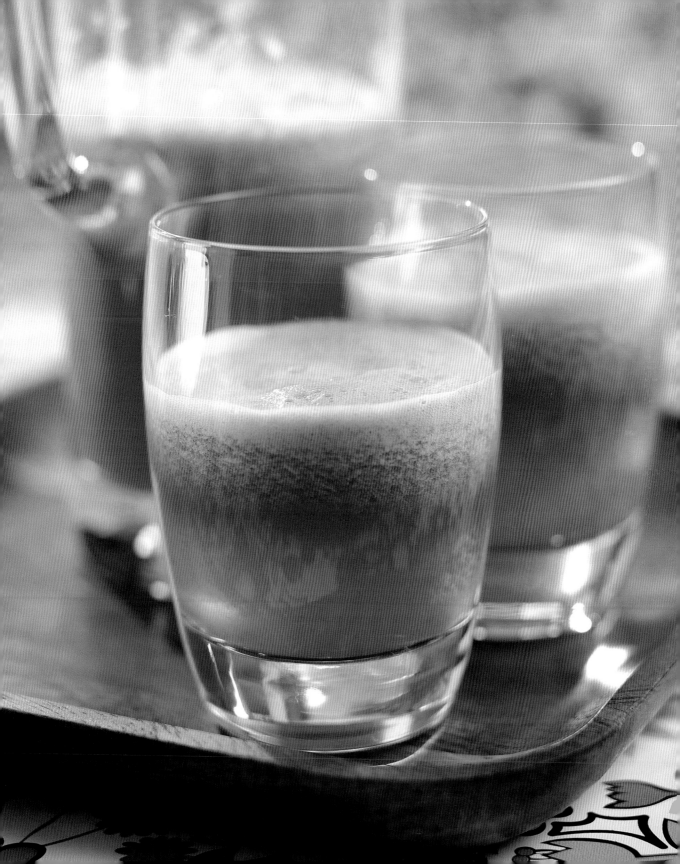

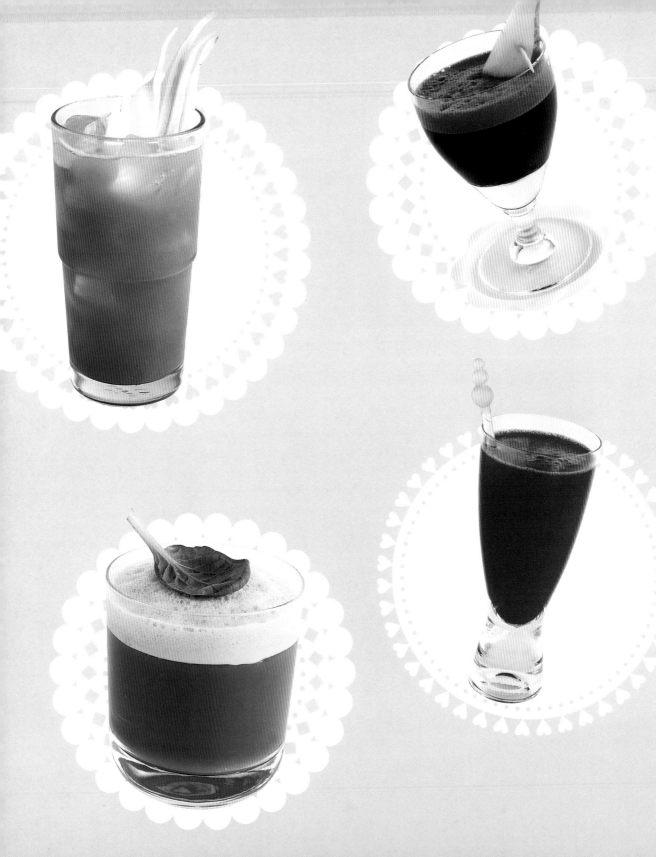

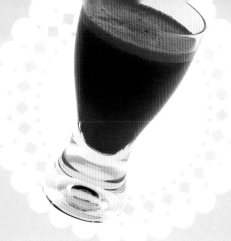

VITAL
VEGGIES

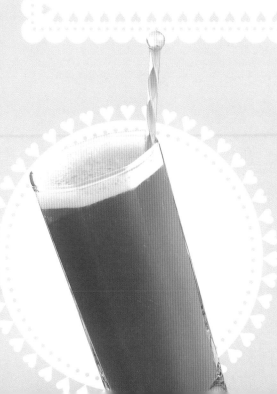

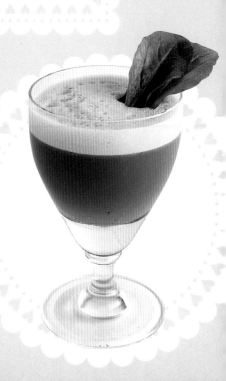

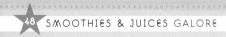

BRILLIANT GREENS

BROCCOLI, ORANGE, SPINACH, CELERY & KELP

The brassica family, which includes broccoli and spinach,
offers a wealth of nutrients. Here, they are combined in a
surprisingly creamy, mild juice, which is full of vitamin C,
iron and beta-carotene and will protect your whole system.

MAKES 1 GLASS

100g broccoli
1 orange
70g baby spinach
1 celery stick
1 teaspoon kelp

1. Roughly chop the broccoli, then peel the orange and divide the flesh into segments.

2. Press the spinach through a juicer, followed by the celery, broccoli and, finally, the orange. Stir the kelp into the juice, then pour into a glass and serve immediately.

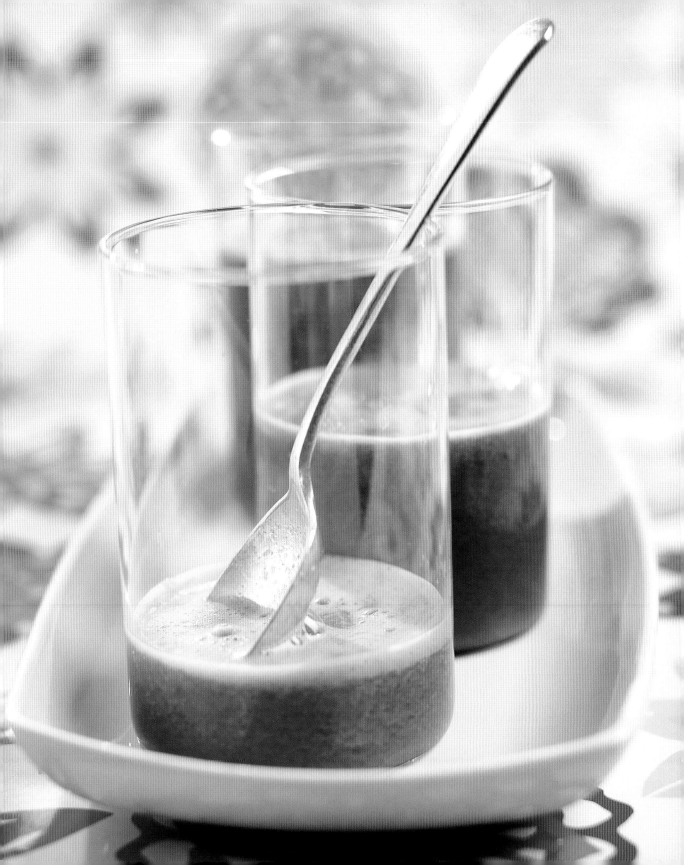

GREEN HOTHOUSE

BROCCOLI, APPLE, SPINACH & HORSERADISH

Fiery horseradish adds a certain bite to this surprisingly mild, sweet juice
and helps to clear the sinuses if you're feeling congested. Sugary apples
offer an instant energy hit, whereas baby spinach and broccoli contain anti-
oxidants to boost your immune system. Spinach also contains zeaxanthin
and lutein, which are thought to protect the eyes against ageing.

MAKES 1 GLASS

150g broccoli
1 1/2 apples
120g baby spinach, plus an extra
   leaf to decorate
3/4 teaspoon grated horseradish

1. Roughly chop the broccoli and apples. Press the spinach leaves through
a juicer, followed by the broccoli and apples.
2. Stir the grated horseradish into the juice and pour into a glass.
Decorate with a baby spinach leaf and serve immediately.

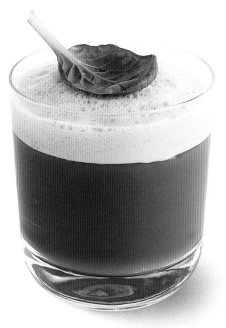

JUICE TIP
*You can alter the
proportions of broccoli and
spinach if you like. They both
produce wonderfully mild juices and
are equally beneficial to your health.
And if you prefer a pepper-free
juice, you can leave out the
horseradish too.*

RED ALERT

RED PEPPER, PINEAPPLE & BEETROOT

Strangely, this energizing blend of vegetables and pineapple has a definite
hint of strawberries in its flavour. The natural fruit sugars give a great
energy boost, while hefty doses of beta-carotene, vitamin C and other
health-giving nutrients and phytochemicals will have you firing on all
cylinders in no time.

MAKES 1 TALL GLASS

1 red pepper
¼ large pineapple (about 450g)
¼ beetroot, scrubbed

1. Cut the pepper in half, remove the seeds, white pith and stalk and
then cut the flesh into chunks. Cut the skin from the pineapple, remove
the central core and cut the flesh into
rough chunks.

2. Press the pepper, pineapple and beetroot
through the juicer, then pour into a tall
glass and serve immediately.

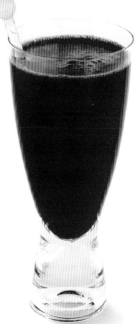

WAKE-UP CALL

CARROT, KIWIFRUIT, YELLOW PEPPER, GINGER & LEMON

Wake up and get going with this fresh and zingy juice. It offers
instant energy, essential health-promoting nutrients and
fabulous flavour.

MAKES 1 GLASS

2 carrots, trimmed
1 kiwifruit
$\frac{1}{2}$ yellow pepper
2.5cm piece of fresh root ginger
1 tablespoon chopped fresh parsley
Juice of $\frac{1}{4}$ lemon

1. Chop the carrots roughly. Peel the kiwifruit and divide into quarters. Remove the seeds, white pith and stalk from the pepper and roughly chop the flesh.

2. Press the ginger and parsley through a juicer, followed by the carrots, kiwifruit and pepper. Stir the juice, squeeze in lemon juice to taste, then pour into a glass and serve immediately.

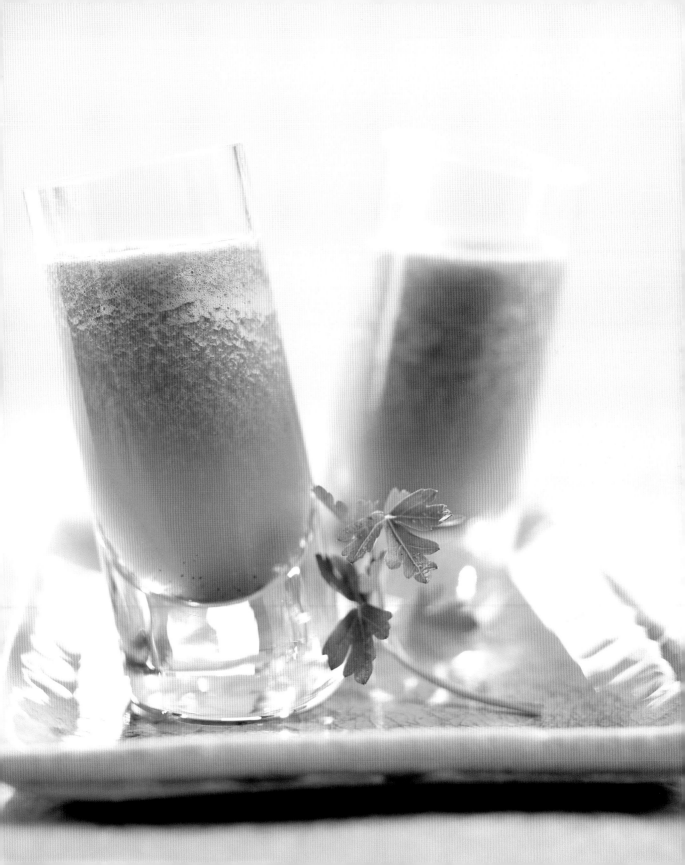

GALLOPING GARLIC

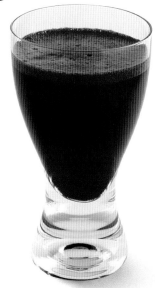

ORANGE, TOMATO, BEETROOT, GARLIC & CELERY

You need only a small glass of this nutrient-rich, blood-red tonic to put your body to rights. Peppery, sweet, sharp, rich and garlicky – sip it slowly to really appreciate the flavours. Beetroot is a great detoxifier and has long been used as a blood fortifier in traditional medicine, whereas celery is valued for its cleansing properties. Garlic has natural anti-bacterial and antifungal properties and adds a delicious bite.

MAKES **1 SMALL GLASS**

½ orange
1 tomato
1 large beetroot
1 garlic clove, peeled
1 celery stick

1. Remove the peel from the orange and chop the tomato and beetroot into rough chunks.

2. Press the garlic through a juicer, followed by the orange, beetroot, tomato, and celery. Stir the juice, then pour into a small glass and sip slowly.

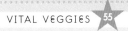

SLEEPY HEAD

CARDAMOM, YELLOW PEPPER, PEAR & ASPARAGUS

Asparagus is well known for its calming properties and is said to promote sleep. Fragrant cardamom, a digestive soother, adds a subtle, warm spice to the juice and the yellow peppers provide vitamin C, which is lost from the body in times of stress.

MAKES 1 TALL GLASS

1½ teaspoon cardamom pods
60ml water
1½ yellow peppers
⅓ pear
100g asparagus

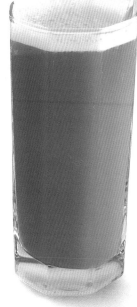

1. Place the cardamom pods in a mortar and crush them lightly with a pestle. Tip into a small pan, add the water and bring to the boil. Reduce the heat to very low and simmer for 3 minutes. Remove the pan from the heat and leave to stand for 10 minutes.

2. Meanwhile, halve the peppers, remove the seeds, white pith and stalk, and roughly chop the flesh.

3. Roughly chop the pear. Press the asparagus through a juicer, followed by the peppers and pear.

4. Strain the cardamom soaking water into the juice and stir. Pour the juice into a tall glass and serve immediately.

TROPICAL TEASER

LEMON GRASS, LYCHEE, MANGO, PAPAYA & GRAPE

This fabulously indulgent blend of mango, papaya and lychees steeped
with the flavour of zesty lemon grass is sure to smooth over even the
most jagged of edges.

MAKES 1 GLASS

1 lemon grass stalk
65ml water
50g lychees
½ mango
½ papaya
90g white grapes

1. Gently crush the lemon grass stalk, then place in a small pan with the water. Bring to the boil, then simmer for 2 minutes. Leave to cool.
2. Meanwhile, peel the lychees and remove the black pits. Peel the mango and chop the flesh away from the stone.
3. Scoop out the seeds from the papaya, then peel and chop the flesh.
4. Press the fruit through a juicer. Strain the lemon grass water into the juice and stir. Pour into a glass and serve immediately.

JUICE TIP
*Don't make this ahead
of time as it darkens on
standing. This doesn't alter the
flavour, but the drink doesn't
look quite as appetizing as
when freshly made.*

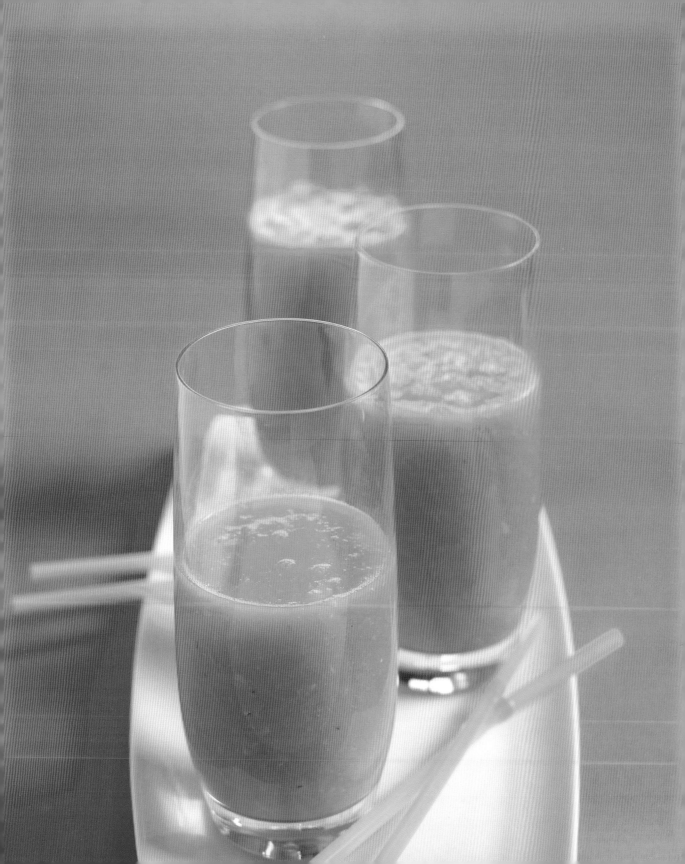

COOL AS A CUCUMBER

FENNEL & CUCUMBER

Calm down at the end of a busy day with a tall glass of this milky, soothing blend. Fennel gives the juice a faint hint of aniseed and is also believed to have a calming, restful effect on the body. In traditional medicine, it is often recommended as a remedy for headaches and migraine.

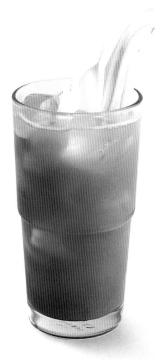

MAKES **1 TALL GLASS**

1½ fennel bulbs, plus extra
   to decorate
7.5cm chunk of cucumber

1. Cut the fennel and cucumber into rough chunks and then press them through a juicer.

2. Stir, then pour into a tall glass, decorate with wedges of fennel and sip slowly.

THE BIG RED

CUMIN, RED CABBAGE, BEETROOT, BROCCOLI & PEAR

Red cabbage and cumin are classic partners and offer a powerhouse of nutrients. The cabbage is packed with disease-fighting phytochemicals and vitamins, while cumin is considered to be a potent, antioxidant super-spice. Drink the juice immediately: if left to stand the cabbage flavour intensifies and becomes unpleasant.

MAKES 1 SMALL GLASS

1$\frac{1}{2}$ tablespoon boiling water
$\frac{1}{2}$ teaspoon cumin seeds
150g red cabbage
$\frac{1}{2}$ beetroot
30g broccoli florets
$\frac{1}{4}$ pear, plus an extra wedge, to decorate

1. Place the cumin seeds in a mortar and crush with a pestle. Add the boiling water and steep for 5 minutes. Meanwhile, chop the cabbage and beetroot.

2. Strain the cumin infusion, reserving the juice and discarding the seeds. Press the vegetables and pear through a juicer and then stir the cumin infusion into the juice. Pour into a small glass, decorate with a wedge of pear threaded on to a cocktail stick and serve immediately.

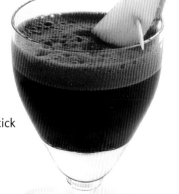

SWEET CINNAMON SQUASH

CINNAMON, SWEET POTATO, BUTTERNUT SQUASH, CARROT & CUCUMBER

Sweet, warmly spiced and utterly refreshing, this calming blend practically forces you to take a step back and chill out. Cinnamon and cucumber help to soothe the system, while the boost of beta-carotene from the orange vegetables will help to protect the body when your defences are down.

MAKES 1 TALL GLASS

1 cinnamon stick
120ml water
75g sweet potato, peeled
75g butternut squash, peeled
1 carrot, trimmed
5cm slice of cucumber

1. Put the cinnamon stick and water in a small pan, bring to the boil and then simmer gently for about 5 minutes. Remove from the heat and leave to cool for 10 minutes. Remove the cinnamon stick.

2. Roughly chop the vegetables, and then press them through a juicer. Stir in the cinnamon water, then pour your juice into a tall glass and serve immediately.

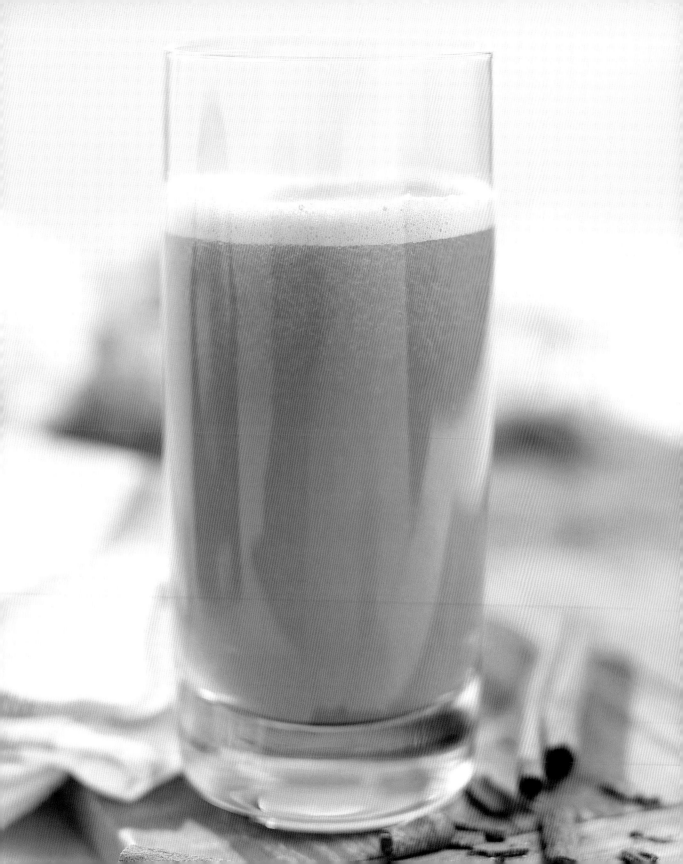

BODY & SOUL

CUCUMBER, GRAPE & MINT

Grapes and mint are both used as traditional calmers, helping to relax the body and mind. The combination of cucumber and grapes is particularly mild and mellow.

MAKES 1 GLASS

½ cucumber, peeled
90g white grapes
1 tablespoon chopped mint

1. Roughly chop the cucumber and push it through a juicer with the grapes.

2. Pour the juice into a food processor or blender, add the mint and process briefly until the mint is finely chopped. Pour into a glass and serve immediately.

VEGE-TASTIC!

APPLE, CELERY, CARROT & TOMATO

This sweet and refreshing veggie juice is packed with healthy vitamins and phytochemicals including beta-carotene and lycopene. It makes a great breakfast juice to get you going first thing, or a pick-me-up when you're flagging later in the day.

MAKES 1 GLASS

1 apple
1 large celery stick
2 carrots, trimmed
Large handful of cherry tomatoes

1. Roughly chop the apple, celery and carrots.

2. Push the cherry tomatoes through the juicer, followed by the apple, celery and carrots.

3. Give the juice a stir, then pour into a glass and serve immediately.

BROCCOLI SPACE ROCKET

ORANGE, BROCCOLI, ROCKET & CELERY

This restorative blend spiced up with peppery rocket is sure to calm you down and make you feel like your old self in no time. Mood-enhancing broccoli and orange blend perfectly with calming celery to make a sweet, pungent juice.

MAKES 1 GLASS

2 oranges
40g broccoli
45g rocket
½ celery stick

1. Peel the oranges and divide into large segments. Break the broccoli into small florets. Set aside one or two leaves of rocket to decorate, if liked, then press the rocket through a juicer, followed by the broccoli, oranges and celery.

2. Give the juice a stir, then pour into a glass, decorate with rocket leaves, if using, and serve immediately.

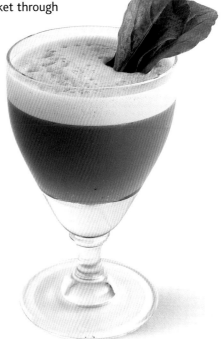

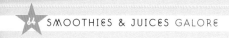

THE BEETROOT & TOMATO POWERHOUSE

BEETROOT, TOMATO & PEAR

Beetroot can produce quite a heavy, intense juice, but this blend of beetroot, tomatoes and pear is light, refreshing and exceedingly sippable. But despite its lightness, it still packs a hefty nutrient punch with beta-carotene, iron, vitamin C and lycopene.

MAKES 1 GLASS

1 beetroot
2 tomatoes
¼ pear

1. Roughly chop the beetroot, tomatoes and pear.

2. Press all the chopped ingredients through a juicer and give the juice a quick stir. Pour into a glass and serve immediately.

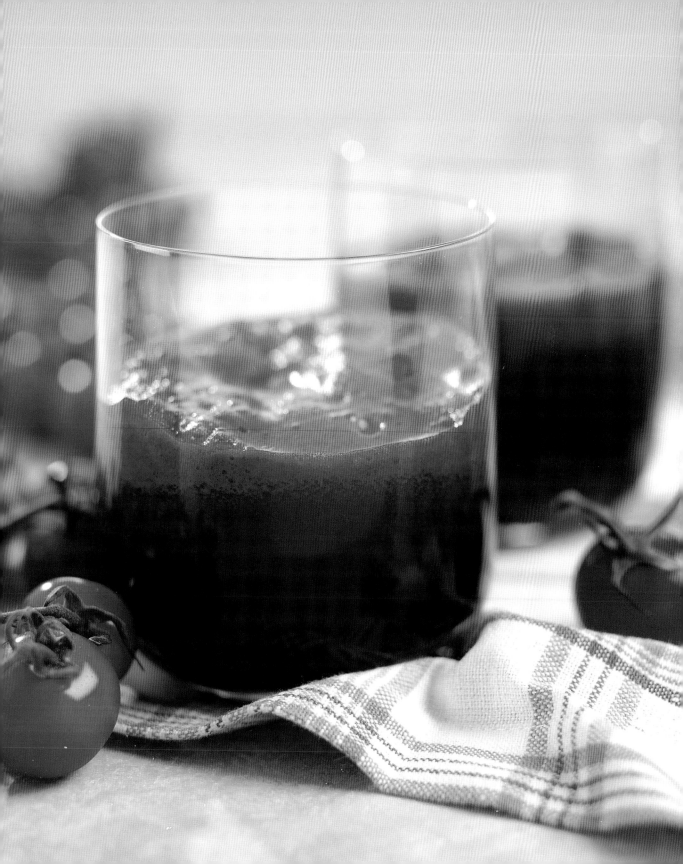

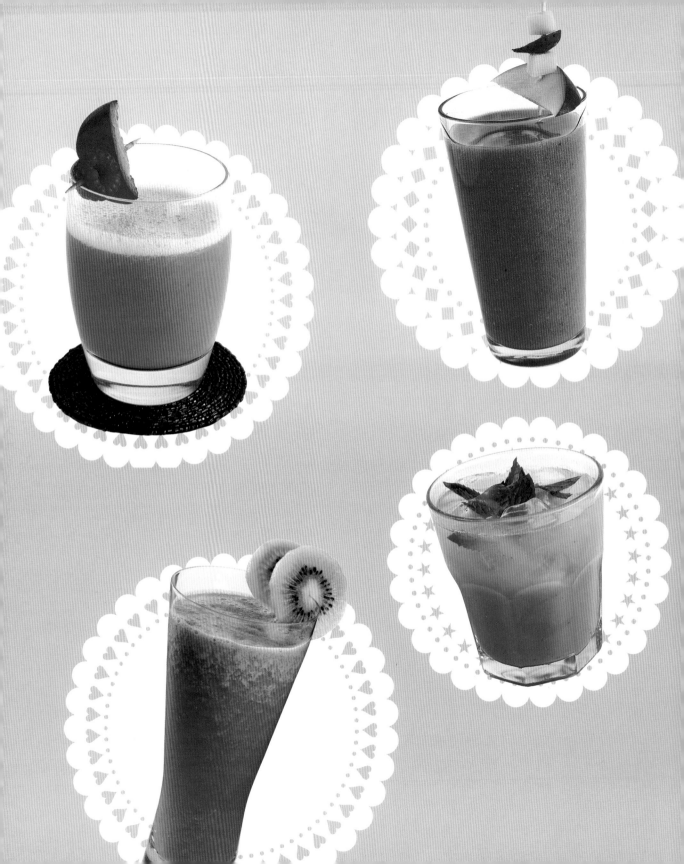

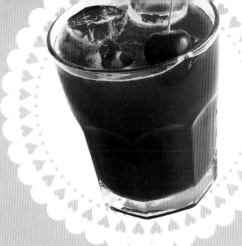

SWEET
& FRUITY

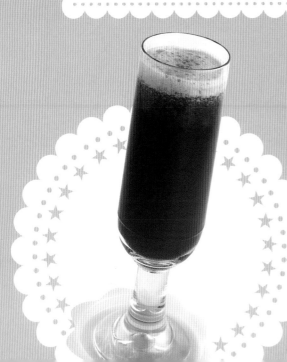

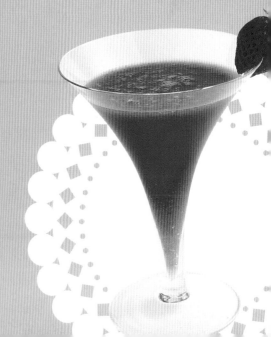

PURE & SIMPLE

PAPAYA, APRICOTS, PEAR & GOTU KOLA

This gutsy juice is a good all-round cleanser and body fortifier. Pears help to flush out toxins, while papayas stimulate the digestive system and apricots strengthen the immune system. Gotu kola is thought to help reduce cellulite.

MAKES 1 GLASS

½ papaya
5 apricots
1 pear
¼ teaspoon gotu kola extract
2 tablespoons water
Crushed ice, to serve

1. Scoop out the seeds from the papaya, peel the fruit and chop the flesh into rough chunks. Cut around the crease of the apricots, twist the two sides apart and lever out the stone. Chop the pear.

2. Press the prepared fruit through a juicer, finishing with the pear. Stir in the gotu kola extract and water. Pour the juice into a glass filled with crushed ice and serve immediately.

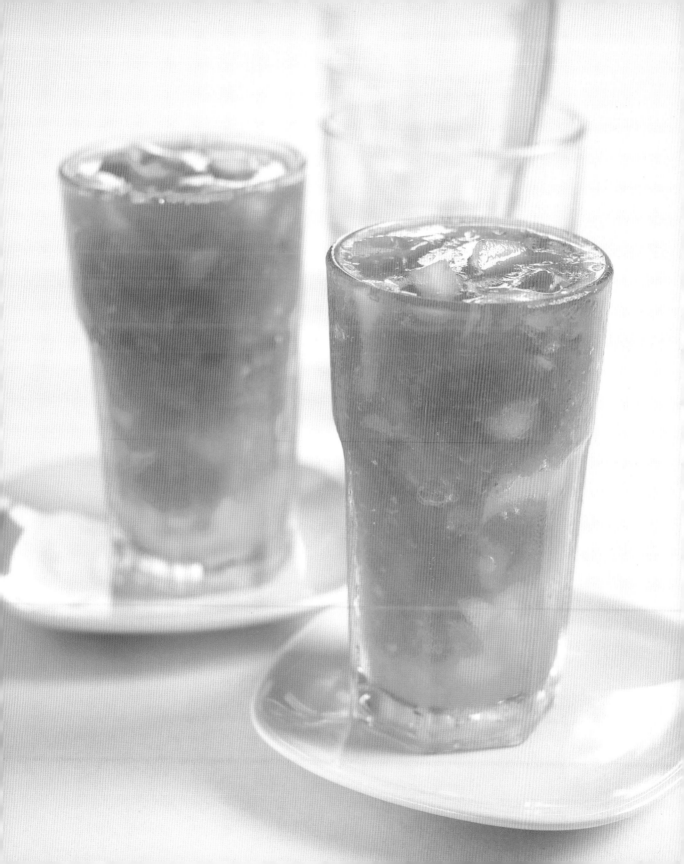

VERY BERRY MELON

WATERMELON, BLUEBERRY & CRANBERRY

Sweet, fruity and unbelievably good for you, this refreshing juice will give you instant energy. Blueberries are an immune booster and, combined with cranberries, are an excellent natural remedy for urinary tract infections. Watermelons offer the additional bonus of lycopene, which is thought to help fight cancer.

MAKES 1 TALL GLASS

475g watermelon
80g blueberries
80g cranberries
Extra berries, to decorate
   (optional)

1. Remove the skin from the watermelon and cut the flesh into large chunks. Press the berries through a juicer, followed by the watermelon.
2. Pour the juice into a tall glass, decorate with extra berries, if liked, and serve immediately.

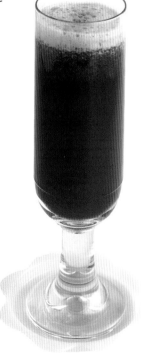

GUARANA PICK-ME-UP

PLUM, ORANGE, RASPBERRY, GUARANA & HONEY

Guarana was originally discovered by the indigenous people
of the Brazilian rainforest. It has amazing energizing powers,
which provide you with a natural boost of sustained energy.

MAKES 1 GLASS

2 ripe plums, plus 1 extra
   to decorate
2 oranges
30g raspberries
$1/4$ teaspoon guarana extract
$1/4$–$1/2$ teaspoon runny honey

1. Cut all the way around the plums, through the creases, then twist apart and lever out the stones. Cut the flesh into large chunks.

2. Peel the oranges and divide the flesh into large chunks. Press the raspberries through a juicer (reserving 1 to decorate), followed by the plums and oranges.

3. Stir in the guarana extract and a little honey, then pour into a glass. Thread a wedge of plum and 1 raspberry on to a cocktail stick and balance on the rim of the glass to decorate. Serve immediately.

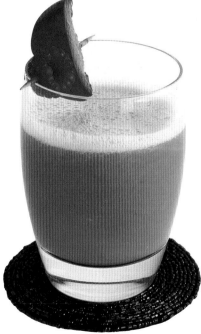

FRUITY CHEER

POMEGRANATE, APPLE, GRAPE, PERSIMMON & LIME

This sweet, sticky smoothie is just the thing when you need a feel-good
pick-me-up. Persimmon gives it a wonderful sweetness and fabulously
velvety texture, while pomegranate, lime and apple juice cut through
with a delicious sharpness to complement the fragrant mint.

MAKES 1 GLASS

¼ pomegranate
½ apple
90g red grapes
1 persimmon
¼–½ lime
Mint sprig, to decorate

1. Scoop the pomegranate seeds into a sieve placed over a blender jug. Using the back of a large spoon, press out the juice from the pomegranate seeds.

2. Chop the apple and then press through a juicer with the grapes. Pour into the blender.

3. Cut the persimmon into wedges and remove the seeds and skin. Place the fruit in the blender. Blend until smooth and creamy. Stir in lime juice to taste, then pour into a glass. Decorate with the mint sprig and serve.

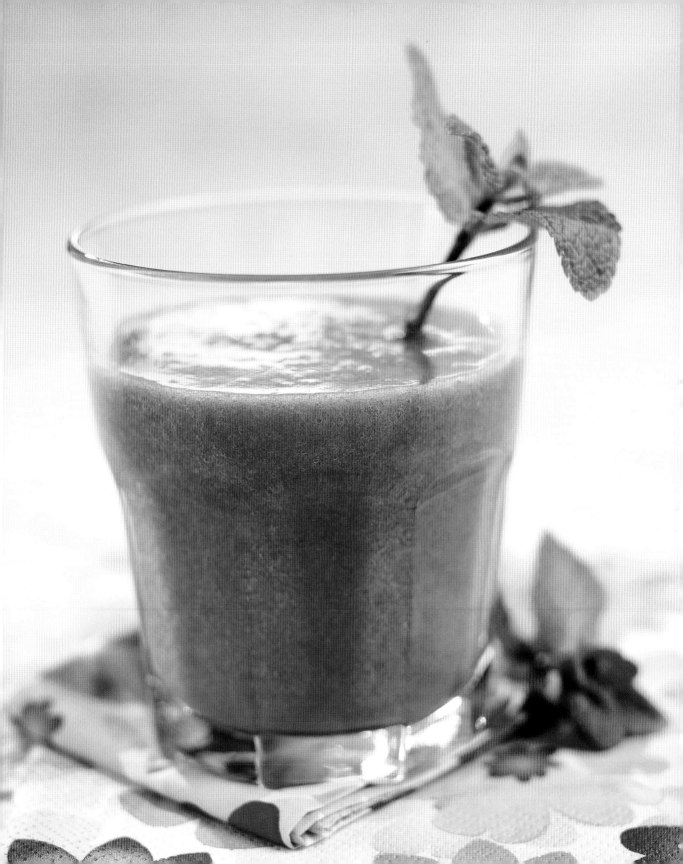

KIWI CALM

KIWIFRUIT, PINEAPPLE, WATERMELON & LEMON

When you want to sit back, relax and indulge yourself, try
a glass of this refreshing juice, which is packed with the
natural anti-stress nutrient, vitamin C. For a truly luxurious
treat, add a scoop of frozen yogurt.

MAKES 1 GLASS

1 kiwifruit, plus extra slices
   to decorate
2¹/₂cm slice of pineapple
250g watermelon
Lemon juice, to taste

1. Peel the kiwifruit and cut into rough chunks. Remove the skin and central core from the pineapple and cut the flesh into rough chunks. Remove the skin from the watermelon and cut the flesh into rough chunks.

2. Press the fruit through a juicer and then stir in a little lemon juice to taste. Pour into a glass, decorate with slices of kiwifruit and serve immediately.

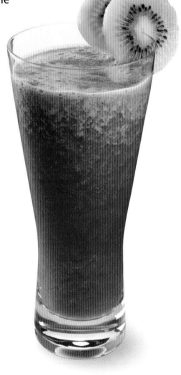

MELON & MANGO DREAMS

MELON, MANGO & ORANGE

Cantaloupe melon is a double winner as it is an excellent source of vitamin A and beta-carotene, and this winning combination with mango will leave you dreaming of tropical beaches.

MAKES 6 GLASSES

1 small cantaloupe melon
1 mango
Juice of 4 oranges

1. Cut the cantaloupe in half. Scoop out and discard the seeds from both halves, then scoop the flesh into a food processor or blender.

2. Peel the mango and cut the flesh away from the stone in large pieces. Add to the food processor or blender.

3. Purée until smooth, pour into a tall jug and stir in the fresh orange juice. Chill thoroughly and serve into 6 tall glasses.

JUICE TIP
You can add sugar to this drink, but if the fruit is ripe enough, you shouldn't need to. For a special treat, add a scoop of orange sorbet or mango ice cream.

MANGO & REDCURRANT RUMBA

BANANA, MANGO & REDCURRANT

The addition of redcurrants gives this sweet, creamy smoothie a deliciously sharp tang that offsets the banana and mango perfectly. If you prefer your smoothie extra thick, use a little less milk and serve your smoothie with a spoon.

MAKES 1 GLASS

½ banana
½ ripe mango
2 tablespoons redcurrants
125ml milk

1. Peel the mango and cut the flesh away from the stone. Place the mango in a food processor or blender.

2. Peel the banana and cut into chunks and put in the food processor or blender with the chopped mango, then add the redcurrants and milk.

3. Blend until smooth and creamy, then pour into a glass and serve.

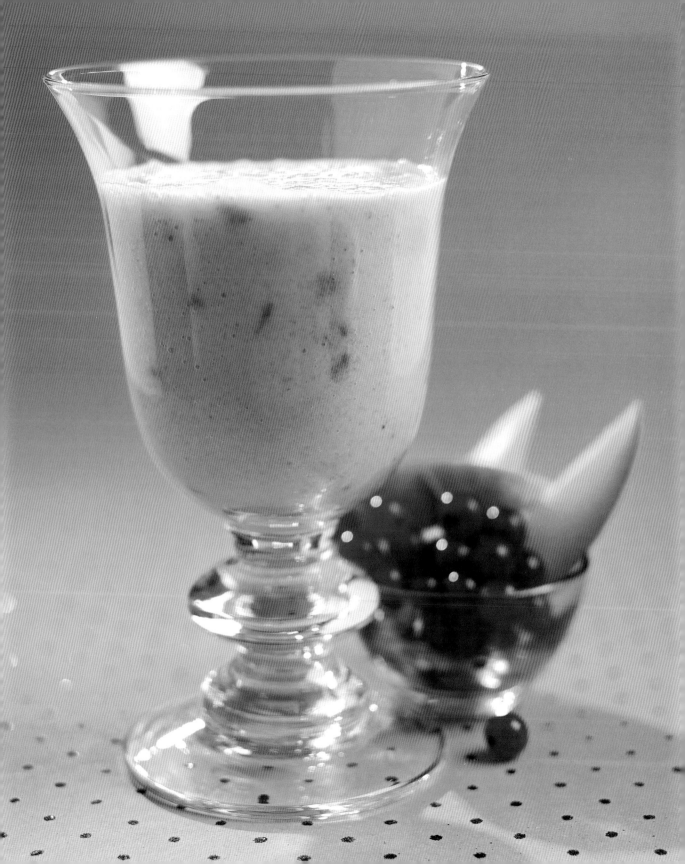

APPLE-NUT ENERGIZER

CASHEW NUTS, ALMONDS & APPLE

If your chosen apple juice is reasonably sweet, you
shouldn't need to add any extra sweetening. Taste the
juice to check and add a little honey or sugar if necessary.

MAKES 4 SMALL GLASSES

150g cashew nuts
150g blanched almonds
120ml water
350ml apple juice

1. Grind the cashews and almonds very finely in a nut mill or coffee grinder. Tip into a tall jug and gradually stir in the water to make a smooth paste.

2. Gradually whisk in the apple juice. The drink will still be quite grainy, so if you want a smoother drink, blend before serving. If you have a hand-held wand blender, use it to improve the texture of the drink.

3. Serve immediately, very cold, in 4 small, chilled glasses.

JUICE TIP
*This also makes a very
acceptable dairy-free ice.
Sweeten it a little (chilling dulls
the flavour slightly) then churn
the mixture in an ice
cream machine.*

MAGNIFICENT MANGO

MANGO, STRAWBERRY & APPLE

Perfect for breakfast or as a pick-me-up later in the day, this thick, fragrant blend is packed with vitamin C, beta-carotene and natural sugars to give you instant energy.

MAKES 1 LARGE GLASS

½ mango
125g strawberries, hulled
2 small dessert apples

1. Peel the mango and cut the flesh away from the stone. Place the mango and strawberries in a food processor or blender, reserving a few small cubes of mango and a slice of strawberry to decorate.

2. Cut the apples into large chunks, reserving a slice, and then press through a juicer. Pour the juice over the fruit and blend until smooth and creamy.

3. Spike the strawberry slice, mango cubes and apple slice on a bamboo skewer. Pour the smoothie into a large glass, add the fruit skewer and serve immediately.

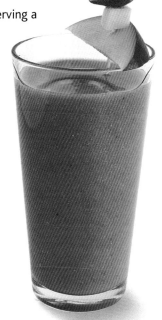

CRANBERRY CUP

CRANBERRY, CINNAMON, LEMON & ORANGE

Sweet, sharp and spiced, this refreshing juice is very good for you – and it has a lovely rich colour, as well.

MAKES 6 GLASSES

450g fresh cranberries
350ml water
1 cinnamon stick
6 tablespoons sugar, or to taste
2 tablespoons lemon juice
Juice of 4 oranges
Sparkling water or lemonade,
   to serve

1. Put the cranberries in a heavy-based saucepan and pour in the water. Add the cinnamon stick and bring to a simmer. Cook the cranberries for 5 minutes, or until they are very soft and have begun to pop.

2. Press them through a sieve into a large jug. Stir in the sugar and lemon juice, and set aside.

3. When the cranberry mixture has cooled, stir in the orange juice.

4. Chill well before serving in 6 glasses, topped up with sparkling water or lemonade.

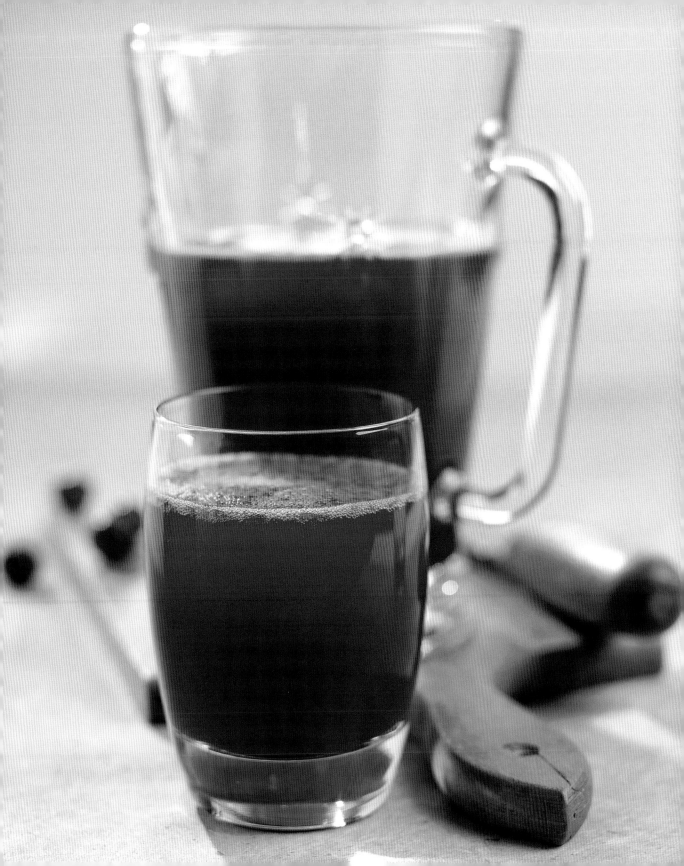

AROMATIC DETOX

PAPAYA, STRAWBERRY, GRAPE & APPLE

One glass of this sweet, aromatic juice and you won't know what's hit you! Its luscious flavour belies its powerful detoxifying effects. Grapes, strawberries and apples are all detox superfoods, cleansing the system and helping to flush out toxins.

MAKES **1 GLASS**

1 papaya
4 large strawberries, hulled, plus
 1 extra to decorate
85g seedless red grapes
½ apple, roughly chopped

1. Halve the papaya and use a teaspoon to scoop out the seeds. Cut the halves into wedges, then peel and discard the skin. Halve the strawberries.

2. Press the papaya and strawberries through a juicer, followed by the seedless grapes and apple. Stir and pour into a glass. Serve decorated with a fresh strawberry.

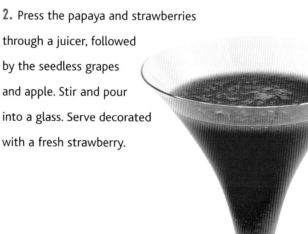

CHERRY-BERRY CLEANSER

CHERRY, BLUEBERRY, GRAPE & LIME

Grapes are great cleansers, and the darker the skin, the more potent their cleansing properties. However, they are often sprayed heavily with pesticides, so it is best to buy organic ones if you can. The juice has an intense flavour, so you'll probably want to dilute it with a little water and serve poured over ice.

MAKES **1 SMALL GLASS**

100g cherries, plus extra
   to decorate
40g blueberries
190g black or red grapes
2–3 tablespoons water
Juice of ¼ lime
Ice cubes, to serve

1. Remove the stalks and stones from the cherries. If you don't have a cherry-pitter, cut around the crease of each cherry, gently prize the two halves apart and pull out the stone.

2. Push the cherries, blueberries and grapes through a juicer and then dilute the juice with the water.

3. Add a squeeze of lime juice to taste and then pour the juice into glass filled with ice cubes. Decorate with an extra cherry.

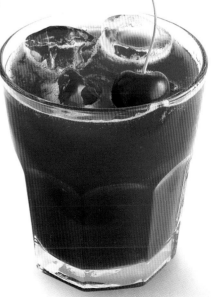

CHERRY MANIA

CHERRY, STRAWBERRY & PEAR

This sweet, sharp, slightly astringent juice will have you up and buzzing in no time. Cherries and pears will boost your energy levels, and strawberries also contain valuable B vitamins. To make a cleansing variation with a slightly milder flavour, try using a large wedge of cantaloupe melon in place of the pear.

MAKES **1 SMALL GLASS**

80g cherries
5 strawberries, hulled
1 pear, roughly chopped

1. Remove the stalks and stones from the cherries. If you don't have a cherry-pitter, cut around the crease of each cherry, gently prize the two halves apart and pull out the stone.

2. Cut any large strawberries in half, then push all the fruit through a juicer. Stir, then pour the juice into a small glass and sip slowly.

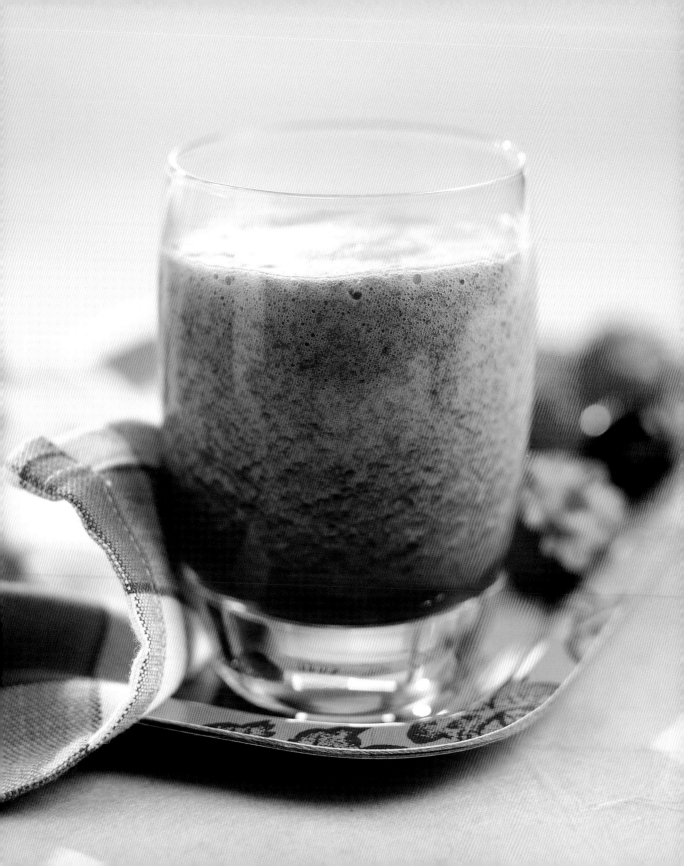

FRUITY JUNIPER SOOTHER

JUNIPER BERRY, LETTUCE, PEAR & BLACKCURRANT

Crisp lettuce and juniper berries give this unusual yet refreshing juice a slightly bitter tang and have calming properties that will ease you into the comfort zone in no time.

MAKES 1 GLASS

$1/2$ teaspoon juniper berries
80ml boiling water
225g iceberg lettuce
$1^1/2$ pears
135g blackcurrants

1. Lightly crush the juniper berries. Place them in a small pan, pour over the boiling water and simmer for 5 minutes. Leave to cool, then strain the juice into a jug and discard the juniper berries.

2. Roughly chop the lettuce and pears. Press the blackcurrants through a juicer followed by the lettuce and pears.

3. Stir in the juniper juice, then pour into a glass and serve immediately.

GREEN GODDESS

KIWIFRUIT, ORANGE, APPLE & MINT

Tantalizingly tangy and refreshingly minty, this luscious
green juice will start by tempting your taste buds before
moving on to the rest of your body to work its magic.
Packed with invigorating vitamins and soothing mint, this
is a great juice to sip first thing.

MAKES 1 GLASS

1 kiwifruit
1 orange
1 apple
15g fresh mint leaves, plus extra to
    decorate
Ice cubes, to serve (optional)

1. Peel the kiwifruit and orange, also removing the pith, and then roughly
chop all the fruit. Press the mint leaves through a juicer followed by the
kiwifruit, orange and apple.

2. Stir the juice and then pour into a glass. Add a few ice cubes, if liked,
and decorate with mint.

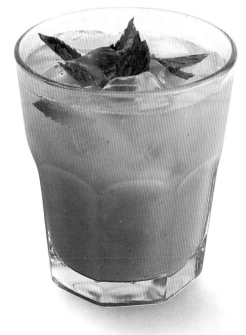

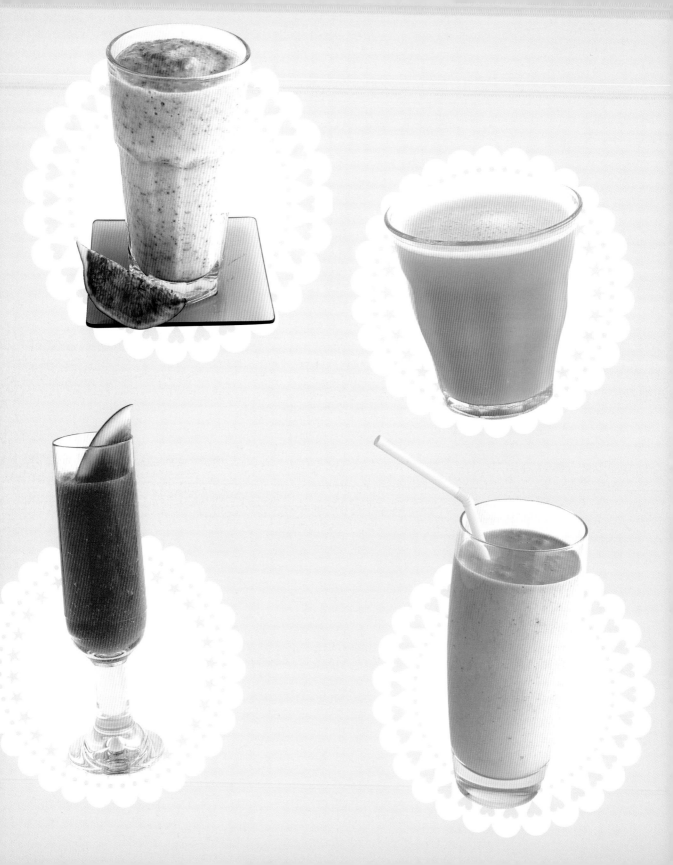

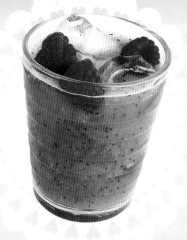

BREAKFAST BLENDS

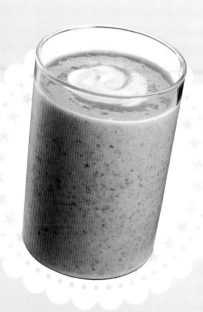

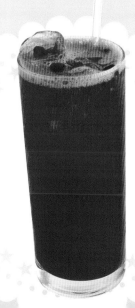

BLOODY MARY

CELERY, TOMATO, TABASCO & VODKA

A fresh, peppery Bloody Mary is the classic 'hair of the dog' hangover cure.

This one's pretty mild with just a slosh of vodka, but it's potent enough to do

the trick without fear of starting you off on the road to another hangover!

MAKES 1 GLASS

½ celery stick, plus extra
  to decorate
1½ large tomatoes
Good splash of Tabasco sauce
1 tablespoon vodka
Ice cubes, to serve

1. Press the celery and tomatoes through a juicer. Add a good splash of Tabasco to the juice and stir in the vodka.

2. Pout the juice into a glass filled with ice cubes, decorate with a celery stick and serve immediately.

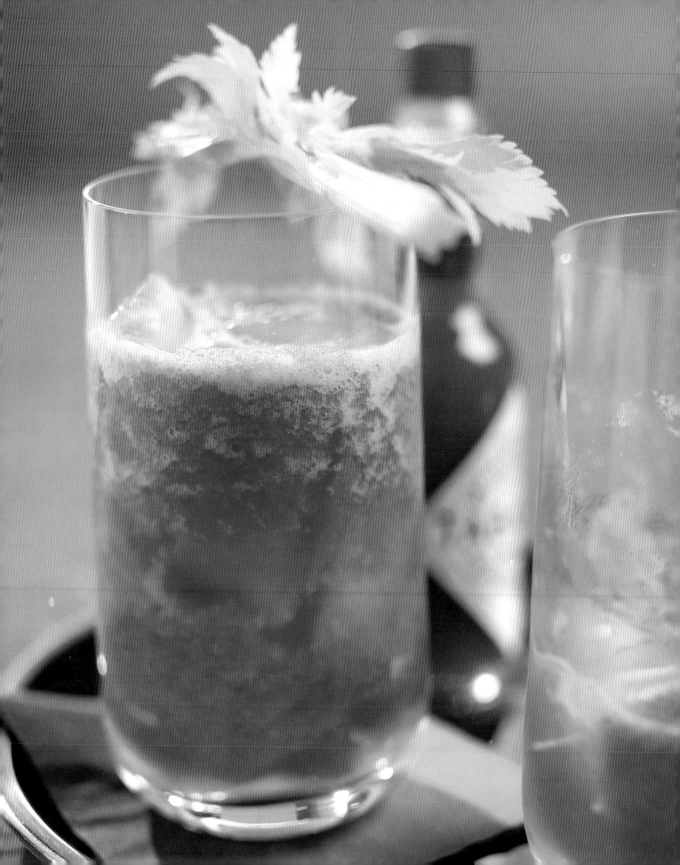

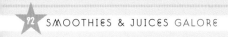

SWEET & CREAMY MUESLI SMOOTHIE

DATE, MUESLI, MILK, YOGURT & CINNAMON

Sticky dates give this healthy smoothie a lovely sweetness without the harshness of refined sugar. The muesli gives it a delicious oaty tang that's mellow and creamy, and just right for delicate early morning digestion.

MAKES 1 GLASS

4 dates, pitted
6 tablespoons muesli
150ml milk
5 tablespoons plain yogurt
Pinch of cinnamon

1. Put all of the ingredients in a food processor or blender, reserving 1 tablespoon plain yogurt to decorate, and blend for at least 1 minute until really smooth and creamy, and the muesli has been completely mixed in.

2. Pour into a glass, decorate with the reserved tablespoon of plain yogurt and serve immediately.

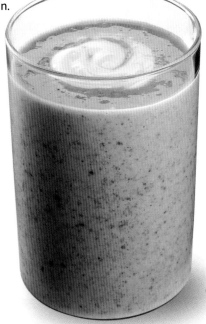

PARSNIP PERKS

YELLOW PEPPER, PARSNIP, BABY TOMATO & RADISH

This glorious yellow juice, with its sweet, mild, refreshing flavour will put a spring in your step. Parsnips are great for the skin, hair and nails, while peppers are a good source of vitamin C and excellent for boosting the immune system. Peppery radishes can help to clear the sinuses if you're feeling congested.

MAKES 1 GLASS

1¼ yellow peppers
¼ parsnip, trimmed
3 cherry tomatoes
6 radishes, trimmed

1. Halve the peppers and remove the seeds, white pith and stalk, then roughly chop the flesh. Roughly chop the parsnip.
2. Press the tomatoes, radishes and parsnip through the juicer, followed by the peppers. Stir the juice, then pour into a glass and serve immediately.

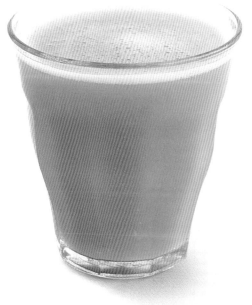

CREAMY DATE & ESPRESSO SMOOTHIE

DATE, ESPRESSO, YOGURT & MILK

This sweet, creamy smoothie has an intriguing, honeyed taste and a caffeine kick that's just right for breakfast. It'll give you the energy boost you need to get you up and going first thing in the morning and have you buzzing with feel-good energy all morning.

MAKES 1 GLASS

4 dates, pitted
3–4 tablespoons cold espresso
4 tablespoons plain yogurt
125ml milk

1. Put all of the ingredients in a food processor or blender and blend for about 1 minute until really smooth and creamy.
2. Pour into a glass and serve immediately.

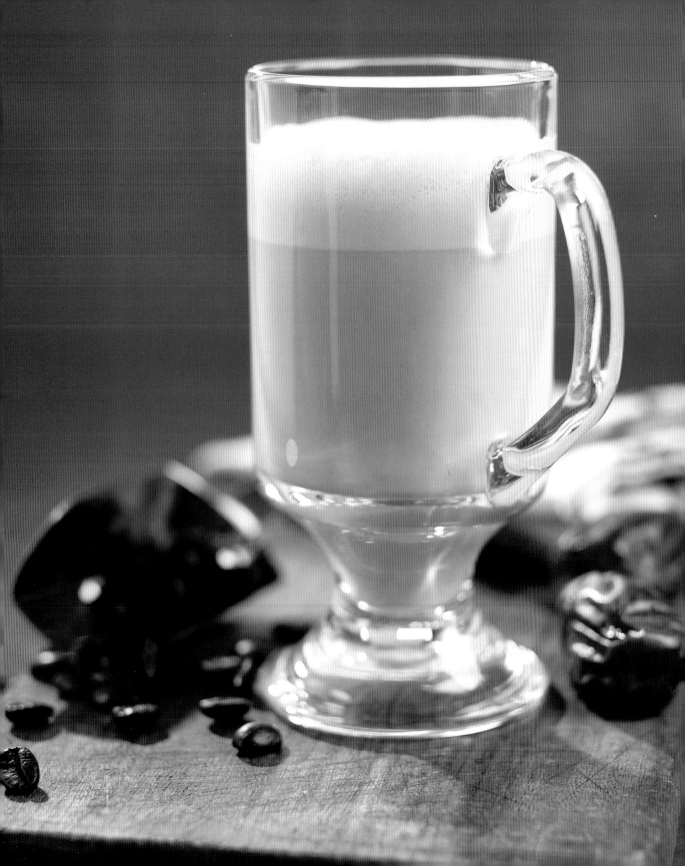

DARK & LIGHT

PRUNE, YOGURT & MILK

Thick and creamy and not too sweet, this makes the perfect storecupboard breakfast smoothie to throw together when you're in a hurry. It's packed with fibre and guaranteed to give you that feel-good energy boost you need first thing in the morning.

MAKES 1 GLASS

6 ready-to-eat dried prunes, pitted
100ml plain yogurt
175ml milk

1. Put all of the ingredients in a food processor or blender and blend for about 1 minute until very smooth and creamy.
2. Pour into a glass and serve immediately.

JUMPING GINGER JUICE

GINGER, GRAPE & APPLE

This tongue-tinglingly sweet and gingery juice is just the thing to perk up your taste buds and get your brain buzzing on those mornings when you're feeling a little lacking in lustre. Just throw the ingredients through your juicer then feel your body rev into action.

MAKES 1 GLASS

1cm piece of fresh root ginger
150g white grapes
2 apples, roughly chopped

1. Press the ginger, grapes and apple through a juicer, and give the juice a quick stir.
2. Pour into a glass and serve immediately.

POMEGRANATE REHYDRATOR

POMEGRANATE, WATERMELON & LIME

This long, cool and refreshing drink is the perfect start to any day. You lose fluid levels overnight and dehydration can make you feel tired and lethargic, so make sure you keep your fluid and energy levels up by sipping this sweet, fruity drink first thing in the morning.

MAKES 1 TALL GLASS

1/2 pomegranate
550g watermelon
1/2–1 teaspoon lime juice
Pomegranate seeds, to decorate
Ice cubes, to serve

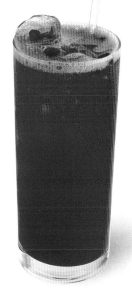

1. Using a teaspoon, scoop the pomegranate seeds into a sieve placed over a bowl (reserving a few seeds to decorate). Press the seeds with the back of the spoon to extract all the juice and then discard the seeds in the sieve.

2. Remove the skin from the watermelon and cut the flesh into rough chunks. Press the watermelon through a juicer, and then add to the pomegranate juice.

3. Stir in the lime juice to taste, pour into a tall glass filled with ice cubes and decorate with pomegranate seeds. Serve immediately.

JUICE TIP

If you're having problems removing the pomegranate seeds, tap the fruit with the flat back of a wooden spoon. The seeds should pop right out into the sieve. Press the skin inside out to remove any remaining seeds.

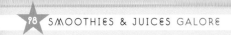

PERKY POMEGRANATE & ORANGE

POMEGRANATE & ORANGE

Sweet and fruity, with that unmistakable citrus zing, a glassful of this refreshing juice is just what you need to wake you up and get your system firing. It's packed with vitamin C for a healthy immune system and folic acid for good cardiovascular health.

MAKES 1 GLASS

½ pomegranate
2 oranges, halved

1. Using a teaspoon, scoop the pomegranate seeds into a sieve placed over a bowl. Press the seeds with the back of the spoon to extract all the juice and then discard the seeds in the sieve.
2. Squeeze the juice from the oranges and stir into the pomegranate juice, then pour into a glass and serve immediately.

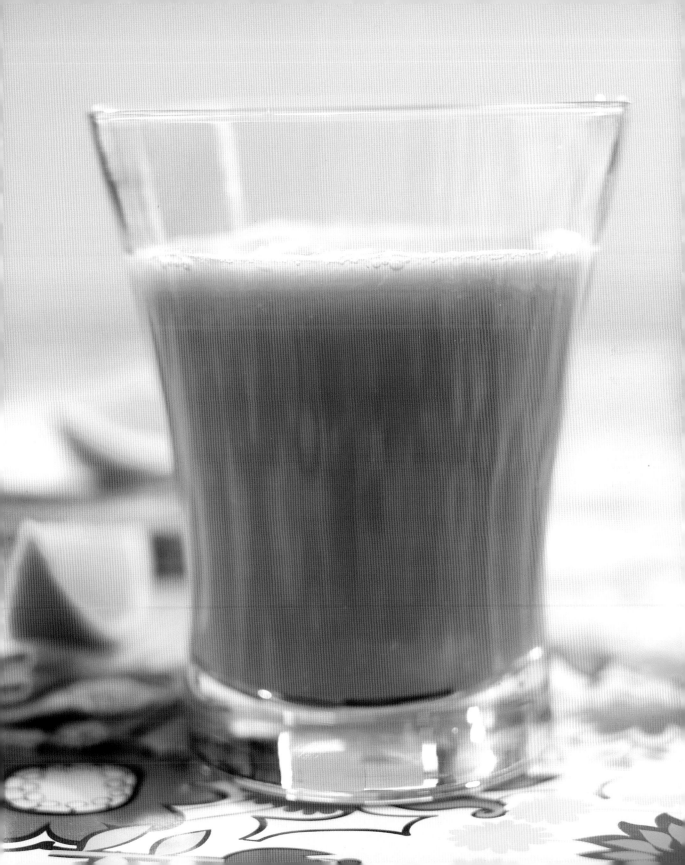

LIFT-ME-UP

BANANA, STRAWBERRY & SOYA MILK

Bananas are a great energy booster, so this mild, creamy blend will give you a real lift. Soya milk and bananas also contain the amino acid tryptophan, which is converted into the mood-enhancing chemical serotonin to lift your spirits.

MAKES 1 LARGE GLASS

1 banana
125g strawberries, hulled
120ml soya milk

1. Peel the banana and cut into big chunks. Place in a food processor or blender with the strawberries and soya milk.
2. Process for about 30 seconds until smooth and creamy, then pour into a large glass and serve immediately.

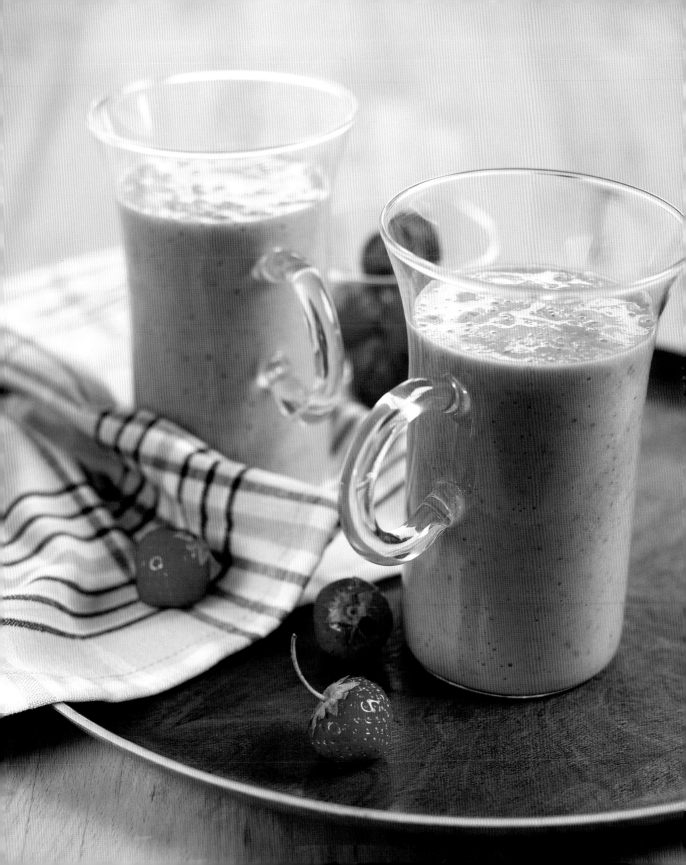

TROPICAL PEP-ME-UP

PAPAYA, KIWIFRUIT, PINEAPPLE, RASPBERRY & POPPY SEED

One glass of this tantalizing combination of tropical fruits and raspberries, packed with vitamin C and B vitamins, and you'll be zipping about in no time.

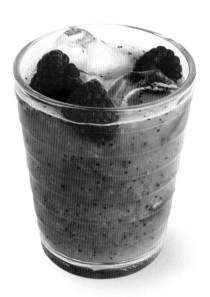

MAKES **1 GLASS**

$^1/_2$ papaya
2 kiwifruit
225g pineapple
30g raspberries, plus extra
   to decorate
$^1/_2$ teaspoon poppy seeds
   (optional)
Ice cubes, to serve

1. Scoop out the seeds from the papaya and discard. Cut the flesh into wedges and peel the skin.

2. Peel the kiwifruit and roughly chop the flesh. Cut the skin from the pineapple, remove the central core and roughly chop the flesh.

3. Press the papaya, raspberries, kiwifruit and pineapple through a juicer. Stir the poppy seeds into the juice, if using, then pour into a glass.

4. Add a few ice cubes, decorate with raspberries and serve immediately.

FIGGY OAT BREAKFAST

OAT, FIG, SOYA MILK & LEMON

Get your day off to a chilled start with this thick, creamy concoction.
Oats are a traditional calmer, and soya milk contains amino acids that
are converted into the mood-enhancing chemical serotonin, so one glass
of this super smoothie will leave you calm and assured.

MAKES 1 GLASS

2 tablespoons rolled oats
60ml boiling water
6 ready-to-eat dried figs
240ml soya milk
1 teaspoon lemon juice

1. Put the oats in a bowl, pour over the boiling water and leave to stand for 10 minutes.

2. Meanwhile, remove the woody stems from the figs and discard. Chop the figs and place them in a food processor or blender.

3. Pour in the soya milk and lemon juice, and then add the soaked oats and any remaining liquid.

4. Blend until smooth and creamy, then pour the mixture into a glass and serve with a spoon.

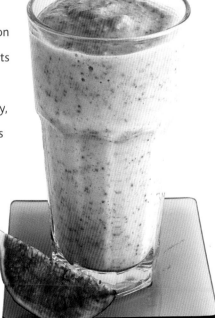

THE BIG WAKE-UP

APPLE, APRICOT, BANANA & BREWER'S YEAST

Packed with apricots, banana, and apples, this creamy smoothie provides a great source of energy. Brewer's yeast is rich in B vitamins, iron, zinc and magnesium.

MAKES 1 GLASS

2 apples
5 apricots
1 banana
1 tablespoon brewer's yeast

1. Roughly chop the apples and press through a juicer reserving a couple of slices to decorate, if liked. Pour the juice into a food processor or blender. Cut around the crease of the apricots, twist the two halves apart and lever out the stones. Add the apricots to the juice.

2. Peel the banana and cut into chunks. Add to the food processor or blender with the brewer's yeast, then blend until smooth and creamy. Pour into a glass, decorate with the reserved slices of apples, if using, and serve.

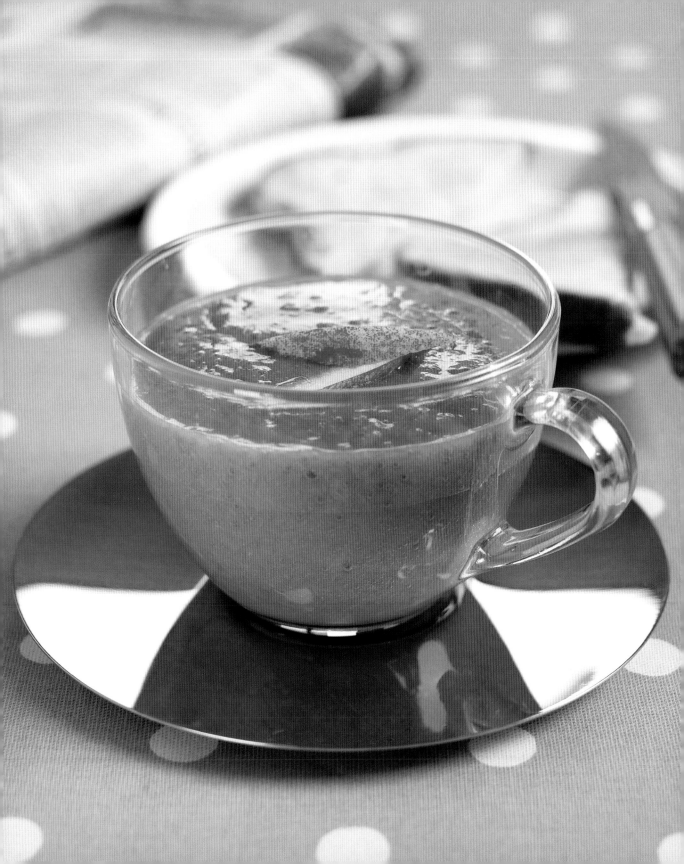

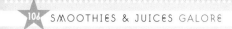
MELLOW MORNING

BANANA, PEANUT BUTTER, WHEATGERM, HONEY & SOYA MILK

Sip this fabulously creamy, frothy smoothie at the start of the day and feel your mood pick up almost immediately. Bananas, peanut butter, wheatgerm and soya milk all contain nutrients that help to calm and lift the spirits making this the perfect choice to start your weekend.

MAKES **1 TALL GLASS**

1 ripe banana
1½ tablespoons peanut butter
1 tablespoon wheatgerm
1 teaspoon clear honey
240ml soya milk

1. Peel the banana and break it into large chunks, then put in a food processor or blender with the peanut butter, wheatgerm, honey and soya milk.

2. Blend for about 1 minute until smooth and frothy. Pour into a tall glass and sip slowly.

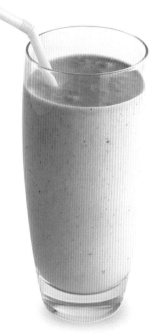

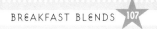

PEACHY SMOOTH

PEACH, WATERMELON & STRAWBERRY

This sweet, fruity juice tastes like a real indulgence, but it's got saintly properties too. Watermelons have a high water content that helps to flush out toxins from the system, but for an extra hit of kidney-boosting potassium, leave the seeds in the fruit as well.

MAKES **1 TALL GLASS**

2 peaches
250g watermelon, plus an extra
    slice to decorate
3 strawberries

1. Place the peaches in a bowl, pour over boiling water and leave to stand for 30 seconds. Drain and then peel away the skins. Cut around the crease of the peach and then twist the two sides apart and lever out the stone.

2. Remove the skin from the watermelon, then roughly chop all the fruit and place in a food processor or blender. Purée for about 30 seconds until the mixture is smooth, then pour into a tall glass, decorate with a slice of melon and serve immediately.

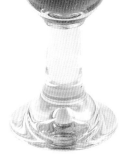

TROPICAL BREEZE

PINEAPPLE, MANGO, SATSUMA & LIME

Fragrant mango, zingy pineapple and zesty lime juice combine to make an enlivening tropical juice-boost. Packed with vitamins and phytochemicals, this makes a perfect breakfast juice or pick-me-up later in the day when you just need to keep going.

MAKES **1 GLASS**

4cm slice of pineapple (about 350g)
$\frac{1}{2}$ mango
1 satsuma, peeled
$1\frac{1}{2}$ teaspoons lime juice

1. Cut the skin off the pineapple, remove the central core and roughly chop the flesh.
2. Using a small, sharp knife, remove the peel from the mango, then slice the flesh away from the stone and roughly chop.
3. Press the mango through the juicer, followed by the satsuma and pineapple, and then stir in the lime juice.
4. Pour into a glass and serve immediately.

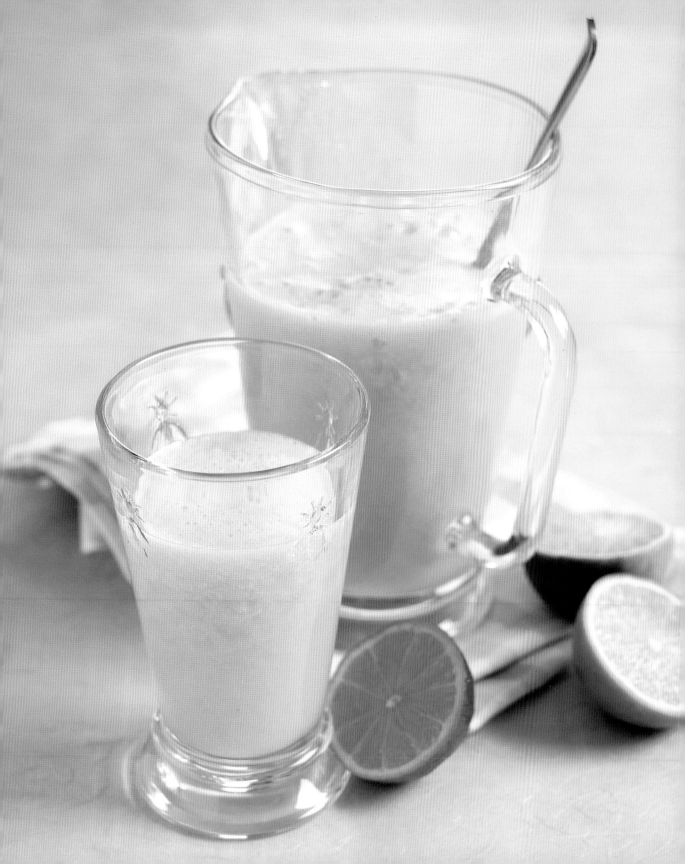

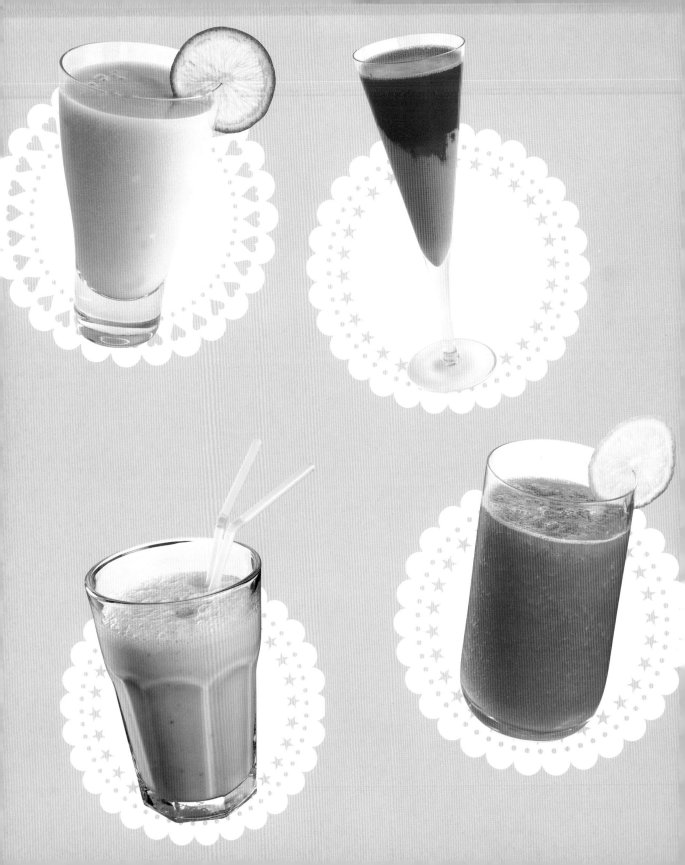

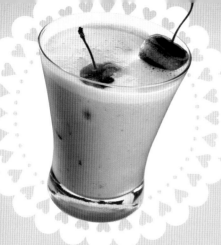

SMOOTH
& CREAMY

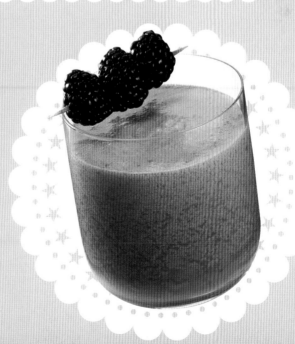

KIWI-TASTIC

PEAR, KIWIFRUIT & LIME

The kiwifruit in this smoothie not only gives it a delightful green colour speckled with its tiny black seeds, but also gives it an almost peppery aftertaste. The sweet, sharp flavour is quite intense so you'll only need a small glassful to satisfy you.

MAKES 1 GLASS

2 pears
1 kiwifruit, peeled and roughly
    chopped
Juice of $\frac{1}{4}$ lime

1. Peel the pears and cut into pieces, then press through a juicer to extract the juice.

2. Pour the juice into a food processor or blender and add the kiwifruit flesh. Blend until smooth, then stir in lime juice to taste. Pour into a glass and serve.

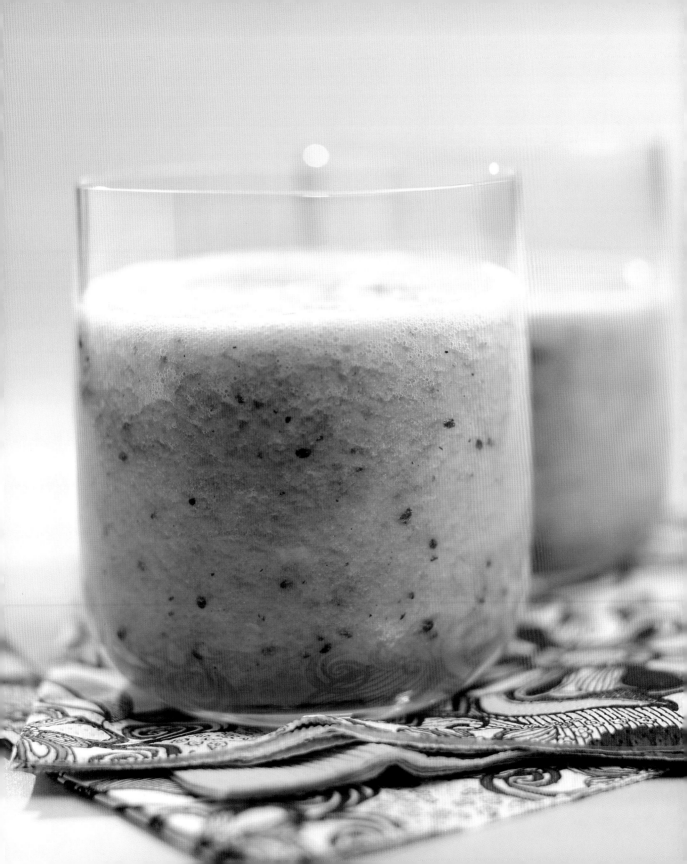

CHERRY BERRY NECTAR

CHERRY, STRAWBERRY, MILK, YOGURT & HONEY

Add a special touch to this juicy drink by making cherry ice cubes – simply pop a whole pitted cherry into each section of your ice cube tray, fill with water as usual and then freeze.

MAKES 4 GLASSES

100g sweet cherries
100g strawberries, hulled
475ml milk
160ml plain yogurt
3 tablespoons honey
Cherry-filled ice cubes, to serve

1. Remove the stalks and stones from the cherries. If you don't have a cherry-pitter, cut around the crease of each cherry, gently prize the two halves apart and putt out the stone.

2. Put the cherries and strawberries in a food processor or blender and add the milk, yogurt and honey. Blend until smooth.

3. Pour into tall glasses and add a couple of cherry-filled ice cubes to each.

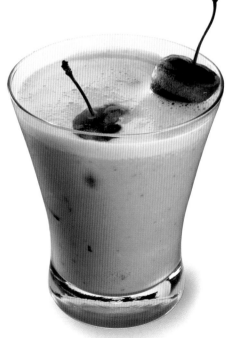

HONEY BEE

BANANA, MILK, HONEY & VANILLA ICE CREAM

This silky smooth drink is very satisfying and perfect for
that mid-afternoon energy slump – the combination of
bananas, honey and ice cream will perk you up in no time.

MAKES 4 TALL GLASSES

2 medium bananas
750ml milk
3 tablespoons honey
1 scoop vanilla ice cream

1. Peel the bananas and chop them. Put them in a food processor or
blender with 240ml of the milk and blend until smooth.
2. Add the remaining milk with the honey and ice cream and blend again.
Pour into 4 tall glasses and serve immediately.

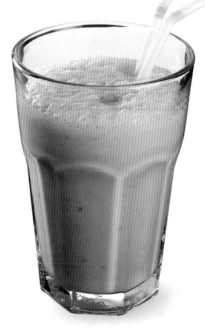

MANGO LASSI

MANGO, YOGURT & LIME

This light, fruity blend originates from India and makes a fabulous refresher on a hot summer's day. Another classic flavouring is banana — so if you're feeling adventurous try a variation using a small banana in place of the mango.

MAKES 1 TALL GLASS

½ ripe mango
150ml plain yogurt
80ml water
1 teaspoon caster sugar
Juice of ¼ lime
Crushed ice or ice cubes, to serve

1. Using a small, sharp knife, remove the peel from the mango, then slice the flesh away from the stone and roughly chop.

2. Put the mango, yogurt, water and sugar in a food processor or blender and blend until smooth and creamy.

3. Stir in the lime juice to taste. Pour into a tall glass with a handful of crushed ice or ice cubes and serve immediately.

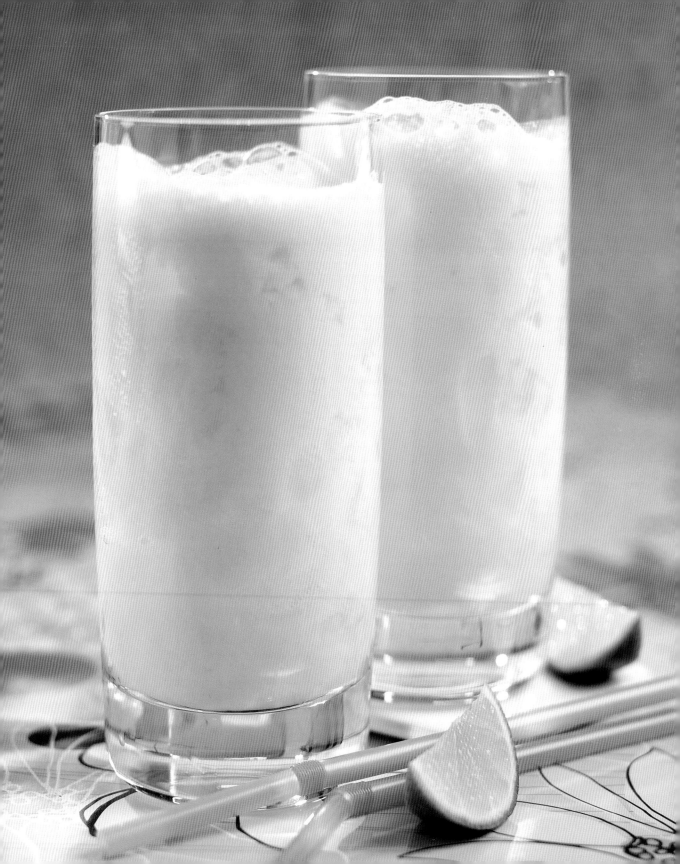

AVOCADO CHILLER

PEAR, GRAPE, AVOCADO & LIME

One sip of this glorious smoothie and you'll assume it's a wicked indulgence, but the great news is that it's good for you. The avocado gives the smoothie a wonderfully rich consistency, while the grapes, which are used in traditional medicine for their calming, restful properties, will help you to chill out and relax. Avocado has the added bonus of being great for your skin so you'll end up looking gorgeous, as well as feeling chilled out!

MAKES 1 TALL GLASS

1 pear
150g white grapes
¼ avocado
Juice of ½ lime, plus a slice
   to decorate

JUICE TIP
*The flesh of avocado
oxidizes and discolours when
exposed to the air. To prevent any
leftover avocado turning brown,
squeeze lemon juice over the
exposed flesh and cover
tightly with clingfilm. Use
within 1 or 2 days.*

1. Roughly chop the pear and then press through a juicer with the grapes. Pour the juice into a food processor or blender.
2. Scoop the avocado flesh from the skin, roughly chop and add to the pear and grape juice. Blend until smooth and creamy.
3. Stir in lime juice to taste, then pour the smoothie into a tall glass, decorate with a slice of lime and serve immediately.

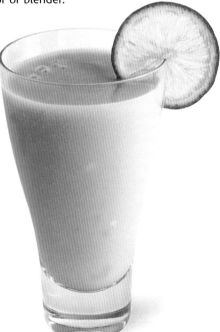

SCARLET FEVER

BEETROOT, ORANGE & YOGURT

A vegetable smoothie may seem like an odd idea but it's
so good and offers the perfect combination for relaxation
and restoration. Beetroot is a natural restorative and blood-
builder, while yogurt is naturally soothing and calming.

MAKES 1 TALL GLASS

1 cooked beetroot
2 oranges
60ml live plain yogurt

1. Roughly chop the beetroot, then peel the oranges and divide into chunks. Press the beetroot through the juicer, followed by the oranges.
2. Reserve about half the juice, then add the yogurt to the remaining juice and stir until well blended.
3. Pour the yogurt mixture into a tall glass and then carefully pour the reserved juice over the back of a spoon so that it floats on top of the smoothie. Serve immediately.

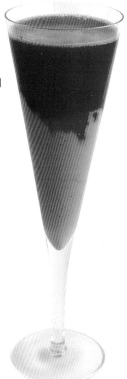

FRUITY DELIGHT

PEACH, STRAWBERRY, REDCURRANTS & GRAPE

Sweet, sharp, tangy and creamy – this is everything that the perfect smoothie should be. For a revitalizing health fix, you can leave out the cream, but for an indulgent treat, stir it in, sit back and enjoy.

MAKES **1 TALL GLASS**

½ large peach, pitted and
　roughly chopped
120g strawberries, hulled
2 tablespoons redcurrants, plus
　extra to decorate
60ml red grape juice
1 tablespoon double cream,
　to serve (optional)

1. Put the peach, strawberries, redcurrants and grape juice in a food processor or blender and blend until smooth and creamy.

2. Pour the smoothie into a tall glass, then drizzle over the cream, if liked. Decorate with a few redcurrants and serve.

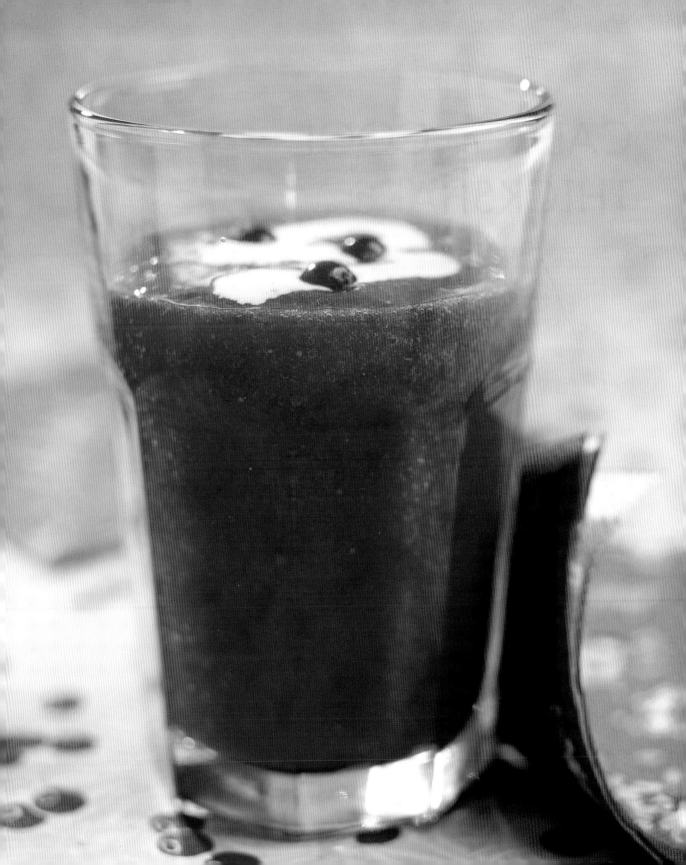

CALM & COOL THICKSHAKE

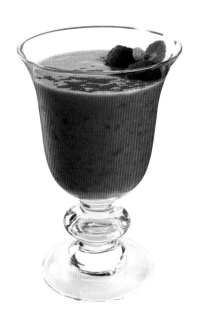

OAT, NECTARINE, RASPBERRY, MILK & LEMON

Oatmeal makes a creamy base for this delicious smoothie and offers the bonus of being a traditional, calming mood-enhancer. Unrefined brown sugar adds to the goodness, being kinder to the body than refined sugar.

MAKES **1 GLASS**

1 tablespoon rolled oats
3 tablespoons boiling water
2 nectarines
40g raspberries, plus extra to
 decorate
60ml milk
2 teaspoons soft light brown sugar
Juice of ½ lemon
Mint sprig, to decorate

1. Place the oats in a bowl, pour over the boiling water and leave to soak for 10 minutes.

2. Meanwhile, cut around the crease of the nectarines, twist the two sides apart and lever out the stones. Chop the flesh.

3. Put the fruit, milk and brown sugar in a food processor or blender, then add the soaked oats and blend until smooth and creamy.

4. Stir in lemon juice to taste, pour into a glass and decorate with a few raspberries and a sprig of mint. Serve immediately.

CHERRY CITRUS MULL

MULLED SPICE, CHERRY & ORANGE

This warmly spiced smoothie is the perfect choice in autumn and winter
when the soft fruits that are classically used for smoothies are out of
season. It's fabulous flavour has a wonderfully festive feel.

MAKES 1 GLASS

1 cinnamon stick
2 cloves
3 juniper berries
125ml water
100g canned, pitted black cherries
1 orange, halved

1. Put the spices in a small pan with the water and bring to the boil.
Reduce the heat and simmer very gently for 5 minutes, then remove
from the heat and leave to cool for 15 minutes.

2. Put the cherries in a food processor or blender, then squeeze the
orange juice over the top. Remove the spices from the pan and add
the water to the fruit, then blend for about 1 minute until really
smooth. Pour into a glass and serve immediately.

PHYSALLIS FEEL-GOOD

BANANA, PHYSALLIS, MILK & HONEY

Rich, smooth and creamy, the physallis in this divine smoothie give it an elusive, hard-to-pinpoint flavour that tantalizes the taste buds. It's fab for a healthy breakfast, but just as good for a feel-good comfort blend when you're feeling blue.

MAKES 1 GLASS

1 banana
100g physallis (about 18), plus
   1 extra to decorate (optional)
180ml milk
$\frac{1}{2}$ teaspoon clear honey

1. Peel the banana and cut into chunks, then put in a food processor or blender. Reserve 1 physallis to decorate, if liked, remove the papery husk from the remaining physallis and add the fruit to the food processor or blender. Pour over the milk, add the honey and then blend until smooth and creamy.

2. Check for sweetness, adding a drizzle more honey, if desired. Pour into a glass and decorate with the reserved physallis, if using. Serve immediately.

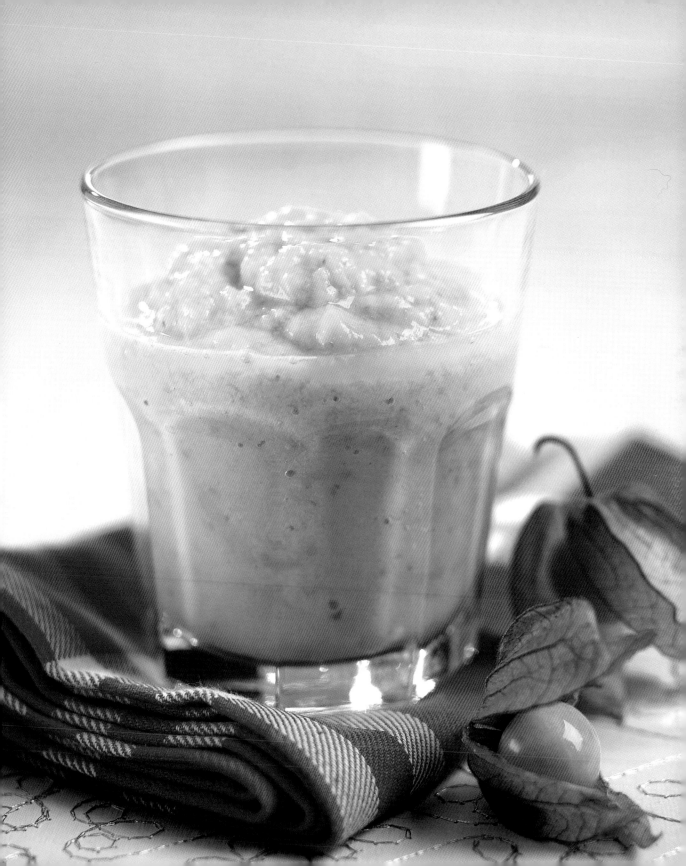

PURPLE TANG

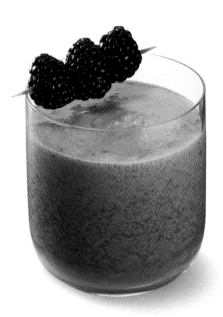

APPLE, BLACKBERRY, CRÈME FRAÎCHE & YOGURT

Although you can use bought apple juice for this recipe, a freshly juiced, well-flavoured apple such as a Braeburn will give much better results. The sharpness of the apples sets off the mild taste of blackberries beautifully, and the addition of crème fraîche gives this smoothie just the right creamy aftertaste.

MAKES 1 GLASS

2 dessert apples or 150ml apple juice
50g blackberries, plus extra to
  decorate
2 tablespoons crème fraîche
2 tablespoons Greek yogurt

1. If using fresh apples, roughly chop the apples and press through a juicer to extract the juice.

2. Pour the juice into a food processor or blender and add the blackberries, crème fraîche and yogurt. Blend until smooth and frothy and pour into a glass.

3. Thread a few blackberries on to a cocktail stick and balance on the rim of the glass to decorate. Serve immediately.

SWEET & SHARP

LIME, YOGURT & MILK

This rich, creamy smoothie has a real kick of intense, mouth-puckeringly zingy lime with a lovely, moreish sweetness. It's great served with a straw so you can sip it slowly and really savour each mouthful.

MAKES 1 GLASS

1 lime
2 tablespoons caster sugar
100ml Greek yogurt
100ml milk

1. Pare the rind from the lime in a single strip to decorate and reserve. Squeeze the juice from the lime and pour into a small bowl.
2. Add the sugar and stir until dissolved, then pour into a food processor or blender and add the yogurt and milk.
3. Blend until light and frothy, then pour into a glass. Decorate with the lime rind and serve immediately.

SUMMER BERRY WHIZZ

STRAWBERRY, RASPBERRY, BLUEBERRY, ORANGE & CRÈME FRAÎCHE

This simple blend of soft berries is one of the easiest, most refreshing smoothies to make and fabulous in summer when fresh berries are at their abundant best. You can go simply fresh and fruity, or add that extra creamy twist, depending on your mood.

MAKES 1 GLASS

120g strawberries, hulled
75g raspberries
75g blueberries
60ml orange juice
2 tablespoons crème fraîche
   (optional)

1. Put the berries and orange juice in a food processor or blender and blend until smooth.

2. If you want a creamy smoothie, add the crème fraîche and blend until thoroughly mixed, otherwise pour into a glass to serve.

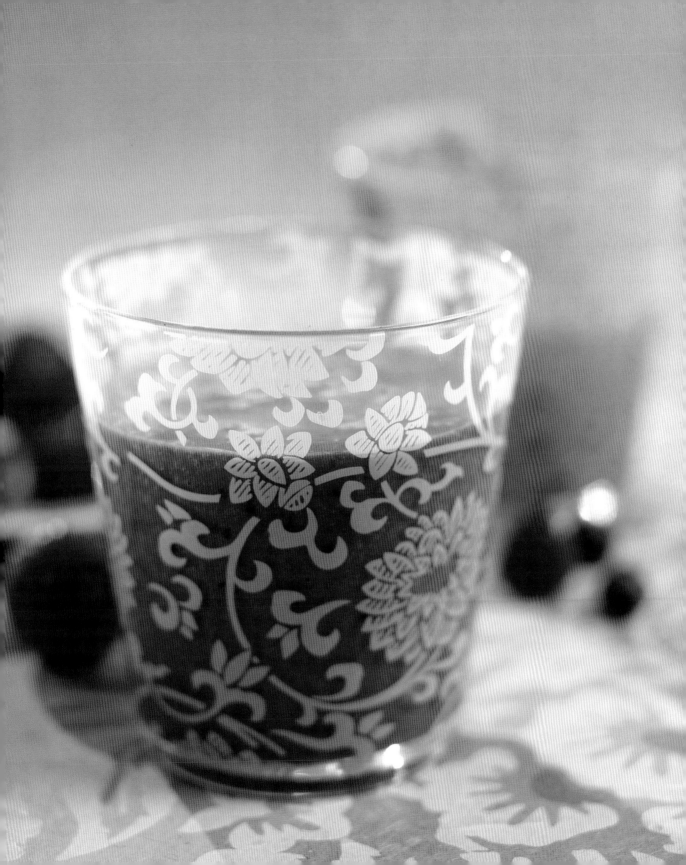

SPICED MELON & PINEAPPLE SMOOTHIE

CINNAMON, CARDAMOM, GINGER, MELON & PINEAPPLE

Smooth, sweet melon, zingy pineapple and scented spiced tea come together in this refreshing, creamy smoothie to make a mouthwatering blend of warm, fruity flavours. It makes a great refresher at any time of day.

MAKES 1 GLASS

1 cinnamon, cardamom and ginger
   tea bag
150ml boiling water
4cm thick slice of honeydew melon
   (about 115g)
3cm thick slice of pineapple, peeled
   and cored (about 115g)
Ice cubes, to serve

1. Put the tea bag in a cup, pour over the boiling water and leave to steep for 5 minutes. Remove the tea bag and leave to cool completely.

2. Remove the seeds from the melon, cut away the skin and chop the flesh into chunks. Put the melon and pineapple in a food processor or blender and blend until smooth. Strain through a sieve to remove any hairy pulp.

3. Dilute the fruit purée with 3 tablespoons of the cooled tea, then pour into a glass filled with ice cubes and serve immediately.

PURE PAPAYA

GRAPE, PAPAYA, MELON & LIME

Sweet and zingy with a tantalizing bite of lime juice, this
simple fruity smoothie is gorgeous enough to give you a
real feel-good hit but with all the goodness of fresh fruit,
vitamins and body-invigorating phytochemicals you need
for good health.

MAKES **1 GLASS**

Large handful of white grapes
$\frac{1}{2}$ papaya, seeded and peeled
$\frac{1}{4}$ cantaloupe melon, seeded,
   peeled and roughly chopped
Juice of $\frac{1}{4}$ lime, plus a slice
   to decorate

1. Put the grapes in a food processor or blender and blend to a purée,
then press the purée through a sieve to remove any skin and pips.

2. Rinse out the food processor or blender,
then return the grape juice with the
papaya and melon and blend until
smooth. Stir in lime juice to taste,
then pour into a glass, decorate
with a slice of lime and serve
immediately.

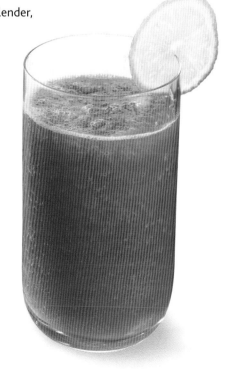

HIGH KICK

APRICOT, GINGER, APPLE, CREAM & YOGURT

Rich, creamy and with the pleasantly sharp tang of apricot and the peppery bite of ginger, this luscious smoothie makes a great treat at any time of day.

MAKES **1 TALL GLASS**

150g canned apricots, drained
1 ball of stem ginger in syrup
3 tablespoons apple juice
75ml plain yogurt
1½ tablespoons double cream

1. Put the apricots, ginger, apple juice and yogurt in a food processor or blender and blend until smooth and creamy.
2. Pour in the cream and blend briefly until combined. Pour into a tall glass and serve immediately.

HOPE & GLORY

PEAR & RASPBERRY

Pear juice is fabulously sweet and offsets the intense sharpness of raspberries perfectly in this gloriously creamy smoothie. If you prefer your smoothie without pips, simply strain it through a sieve before pouring into the glass.

MAKES **1 GLASS**

2 pears
150g raspberries, plus extra
   to decorate

1. Cut the pears into wedges and press through a juicer.
2. Pour the juice into a food processor or blender and add the raspberries. Blend until smooth and creamy and pour into a glass. Decorate with a few raspberries and serve immediately.

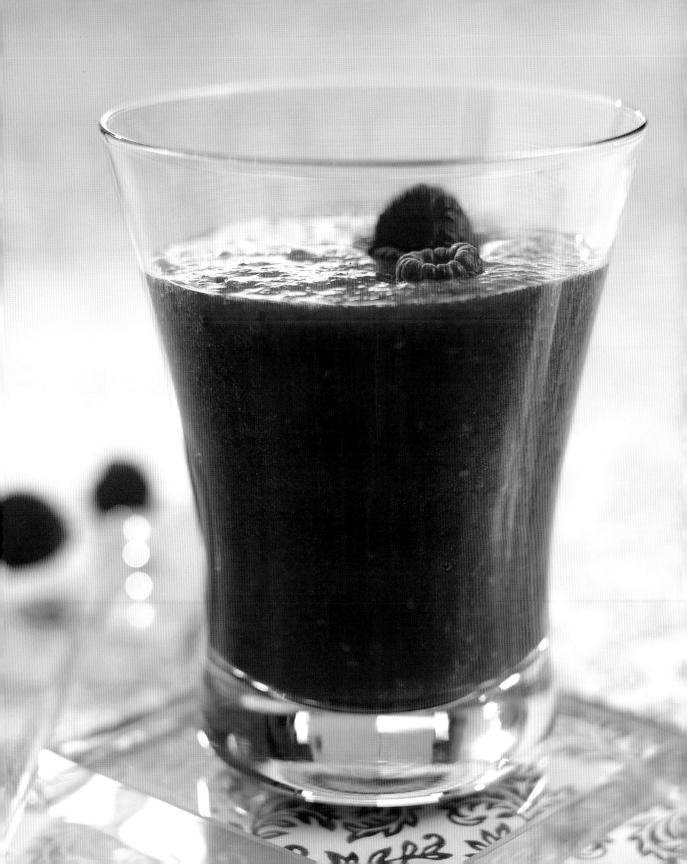

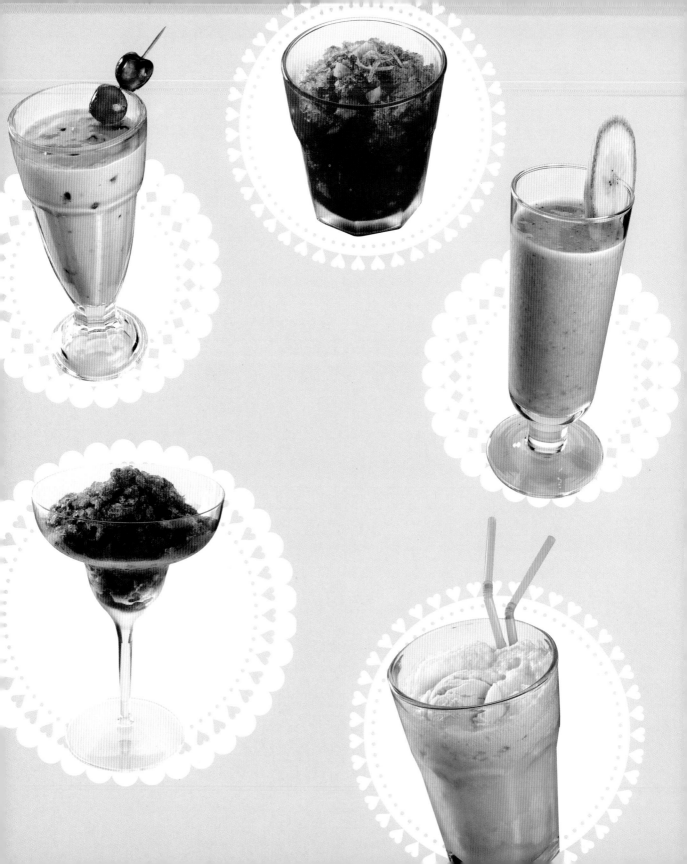

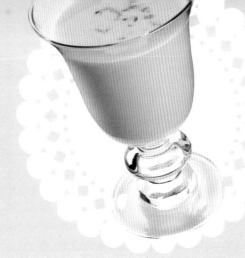

FROZEN & ICED

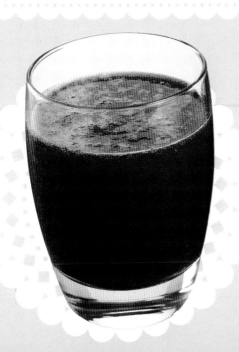

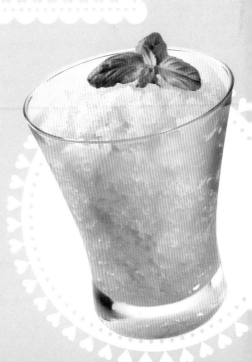

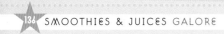

FRUITY FRAGRANT GRANITA

LIME, SUGAR & CLEMENTINE

Sweet, sharp and with an almost fragrant citrus flavour, this refreshing granita is the perfect juicy ice to serve on a hot summer's day. You can use other small citrus fruits such as satsumas or tangerines, but the intense flavour of clementines gives the best results.

MAKES 4 GLASSES

1 lime, plus lime wedges
   to decorate
60g caster sugar
200ml water
8 clementines

1. Using a vegetable peeler, pare the rind from the lime and put in a pan. Add the sugar and water and bring to the boil, stirring, until the sugar has dissolved. Remove from the heat and leave to cool. Remove the rind.

2. Squeeze the juice from the lime and clementines and stir into the syrup. Pour the mixture into a large, freezerproof container, making sure the mixture is no more than 2.5cm deep. Cover and freeze for about 2 hours until the mixture freezes around the edges of the container.

3. Break up the mixture with a fork, mashing it into the liquid and freeze for a further 2 hours. Continue to break up the ice with a fork every 30 minutes until the granita is slushy.

4. Scoop into 4 glasses and serve decorated with lime wedges.

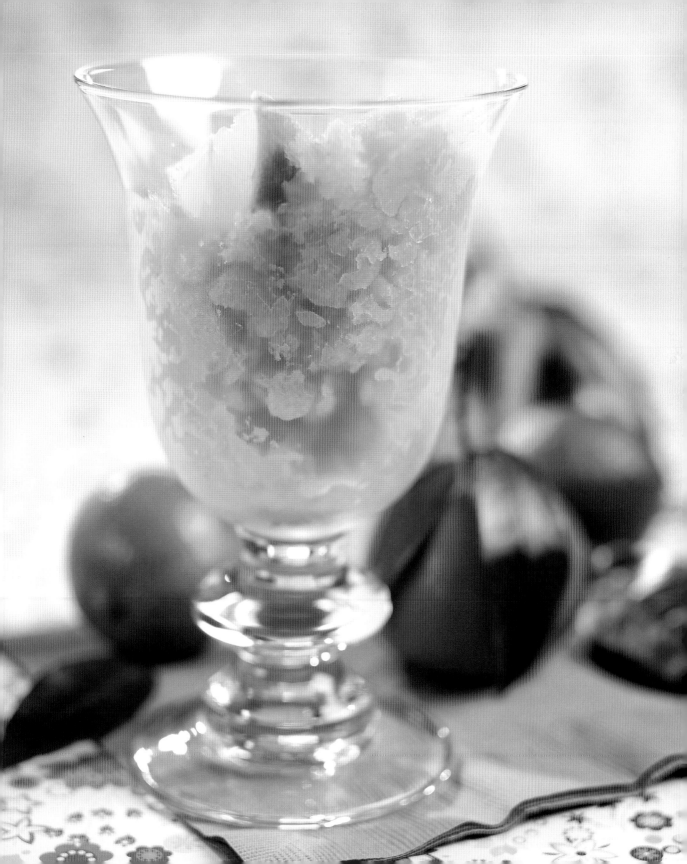

FRUIT ORCHARD SLUSHY

PLUM, PEAR, CINNAMON & LEMON

Rich, sweet and smooth, this silky slush is just perfect in autumn when pears and plums are in season. Although it's icy cold, the flavours and the colour of the slush have a lovely, warming, autumnal feel to them.

MAKES 4 GLASSES

6 plums, pitted and roughly chopped
2 pears, peeled, cored and sliced
40g caster sugar
Pinch of cinnamon
150ml water
Juice of ½ lemon

1. Put the fruit, sugar, cinnamon and 60ml of the water in a pan. Bring to the boil, reduce the heat, cover and then simmer for 10–15 minutes until tender.

2. Place in a food processor or blender and mix until smooth. Strain through a sieve and chill.

3. Stir in the remaining water and lemon juice to taste and pour the mixture into a freezerproof container. Cover and freeze for about 1 hour until the mixture freezes around the edges of the container.

4. Break up the mixture with a fork, mashing it into the liquid and freeze for a further 2 hours. Continue to break up the ice with a fork every 30 minutes until the mixture is thick and slushy. Spoon into 4 glasses and serve immediately.

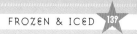

SWEET LAVENDER LULL

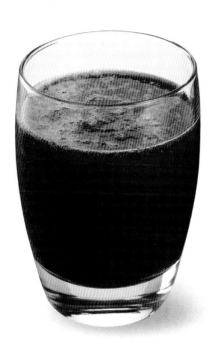

LAVENDER & STRAWBERRY

Icy granita-style slushes are fabulously refreshing when the sun is shining. Make this one on a sweltering hot day, find a shady spot out in the garden, sit back and relax while you scoop up the sweet, delicately scented ice crystals and let them melt on your tongue.

MAKES 4 GLASSES

6 tablespoons caster sugar
200ml water
2 teaspoons dried or fresh
 lavender flowers
475g strawberries, hulled

1. Put the sugar and water in a pan and bring to the boil, stirring, until the sugar dissolves. Remove the pan from the heat, add the lavender flowers, stir and leave to infuse for 20 minutes. Strain into a jug, leave to cool, then chill.

2. Put the strawberries in a food processor or blender and blend until smooth. Strain the purée through a fine sieve to remove the pips.

3. Mix the purée with the sugar syrup and pour the mixture into a freezerproof container, making sure the mixture is no more than 2.5cm deep. Cover and freeze for 2 hours until the mixture freezes around the edges of the container.

4. Break up the mixture with a fork, mashing it into the liquid and freeze for a further 2 hours. Continue to break up the ice with a fork every 30 minutes until the granita is slushy. Scoop into 4 glasses and serve.

JUICY RAINBOW ICE POPS

KIWIFRUIT, STRAWBERRY & MANGO

These traffic light lollies make a great healthy treat for kids in summer – they're particularly popular among smaller children who'll love their bright colours and dinky size. Make sure the fruits are really ripe so the purées are nice and sweet and you don't need to add any extra sugar.

MAKES ABOUT 12 ICE POPS

2 kiwifruits
85g strawberries, hulled
$1/2$ mango, pitted, peeled and
   roughly chopped

1. Using a sharp knife, cut away the skin from the kiwifruits and put the flesh in a food processor or blender. Blend until smooth, then pour the purée into an ice cube tray – there should be enough to fill about four cubes, depending on the size of the tray.

2. Rinse out the food processor or blender. Add the strawberries, blend to a smooth purée and then fill up more cubes in the ice cube tray.

3. Rinse out the food processor or blender for a final time. Add the mango flesh, blend to a smooth purée and then fill up more cubes in the ice cube tray.

4. Freeze for about 30 minutes until the purées are firm, but not frozen solid, then press a wooden lolly stick into each ice cube. Return to the freezer and freeze until solid. To serve, press the lollies out of the tray and arrange on a plate.

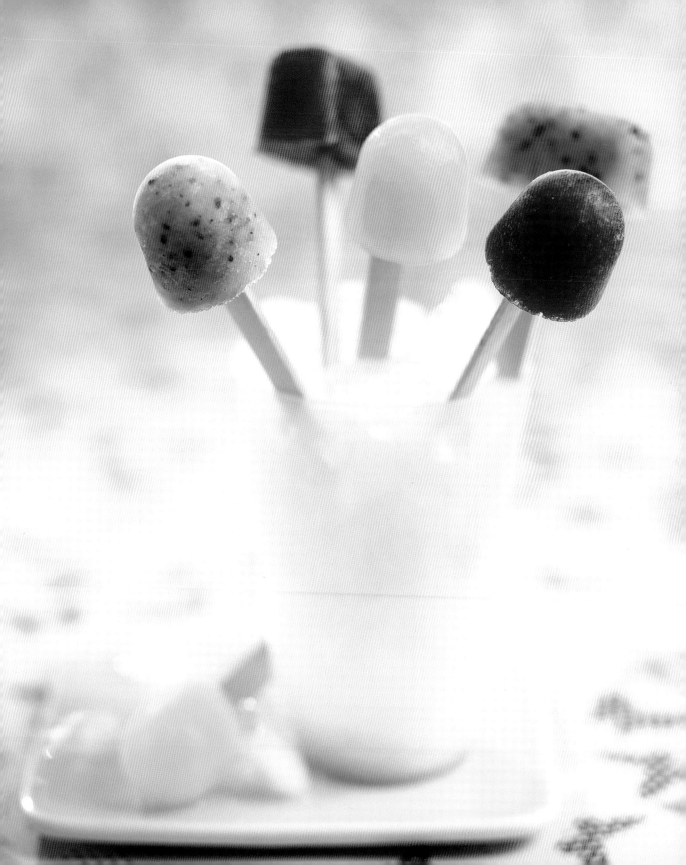

LEMONADE FLOAT

LEMON, VANILLA ICE CREAM & SPARKLING WATER

This quick and simple version of old-fashioned lemonade served with balls of vanilla ice cream is an absolute classic. The sharp, mouth-puckering taste of the lemon contrasts fabulously with the melting sweetness of the ice cream. You can add more or less sugar to the lemon syrup according to whether you prefer your lemonade sharper or sweeter.

MAKES **1 TALL GLASS**

Juice of ¹/₂ lemon
1¹/₂–2 teaspoons caster sugar
2 scoops of vanilla ice cream
Sparkling water
Fresh mint leaves, to decorate
   (optional)

1. Place the lemon juice and sugar in a small bowl and stir until dissolved.

2. Put the ice cream into a tall glass, pour over the lemon syrup and top up with sparkling water.

3. Give it a quick stir to make sure the lemon syrup is well distributed, then decorate with mint leaves, if liked, and serve immediately.

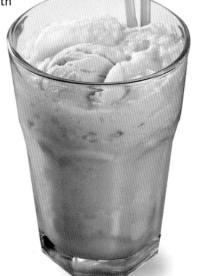

STRAWBERRIES & CREAM

STRAWBERRY, YOGURT & VANILLA ICE CREAM

Icy cold and thick with ice cream, nothing beats a classic like a strawberry milkshake. This version made with rich and creamy Greek yogurt is particularly good, combining the sweetness of the ice cream with the natural astringency of the strawberries and yogurt.

MAKES **1 TALL GLASS**

180g strawberries, hulled
125ml Greek yogurt
2 scoops of vanilla ice cream

1. Slice one strawberry and reserve to decorate. Put the rest in a food processor or blender with the Greek yogurt and 1 scoop of the ice cream and blend until smooth and creamy.

2. Pour the mixture into a tall glass, add the second scoop of ice cream, decorate with the sliced strawberry and serve immediately.

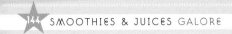

CHERRY CHOC SHAKE

CHERRY, YOGURT, MILK & CHOCOLATE ICE CREAM

Cherries and chocolate are a classic combination and no better than here in this rich creamy shake topped off with dark chocolate ice cream and melting chocolate curls. Look out for a really rich, bitter chocolate ice cream to offset the sweetness of the shake.

MAKES 1 GLASS

100g canned, pitted black cherries
75ml vanilla yogurt
3 tablespoons milk
1 scoop of dark chocolate ice cream
Dark chocolate curls, to decorate

1. Put the cherries, yogurt and milk in a food processor or blender and blend until smooth and creamy.
2. Pour the shake into a glass, add the ice cream and decorate with chocolate curls. Serve immediately.

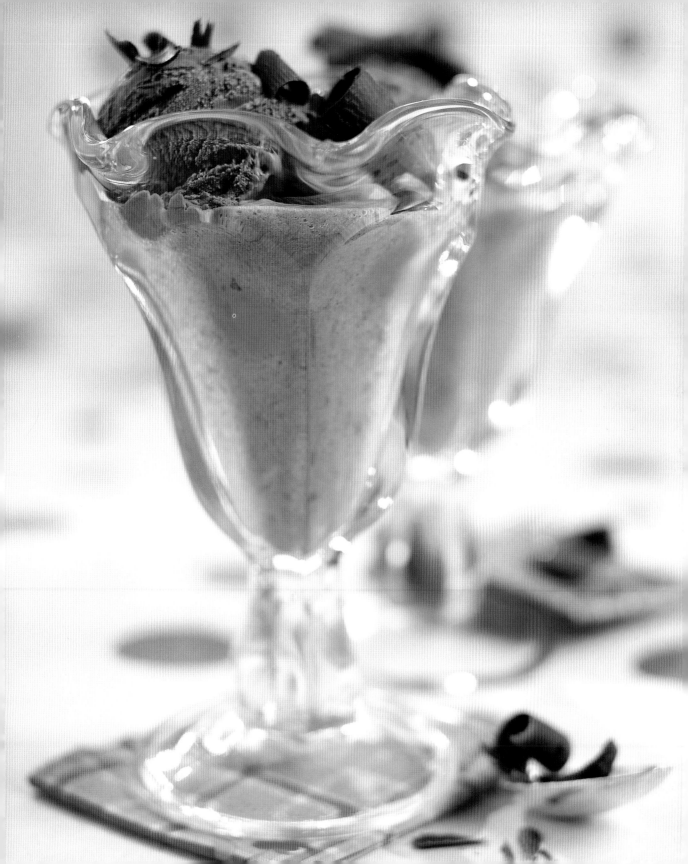

ROCKY ROAD

CHOCOLATE, CREAM, MILK, VANILLA ICE CREAM, NUTS & MARSHMALLOW

This classic combination of chocolate, nuts and marshmallows makes a fabulously indulgent ice cream shake that's all topped off with a rich, fudgey dark chocolate sauce. Kids will love it – but it's perfect for grown ups too.

MAKES **1 GLASS**

50g dark chocolate, chopped
3 tablespoons double cream
175ml chilled milk
2 scoops of vanilla ice cream
2 Brazil nuts, roughly chopped
A few mini marshmallows,
   to decorate

1. Put the chocolate and cream in a heatproof bowl set over a pan of gently simmering water. Heat, stirring occasionally, until melted, then remove from the heat.

2. Put the milk in a food processor or blender and add about two-thirds of the melted chocolate sauce and blend well. Add 1 scoop of ice cream and blend until combined.

3. Pour the shake into a glass and add the second scoop of ice cream. Drizzle over the remaining melted chocolate sauce, sprinkle over the nuts and marshmallows and serve immediately.

RUM-TASTIC SEMIFREDDO

BANANA, RAISIN, MILK & RUM

This smooth, iced treat is perfect as a wickedly indulgent refresher. It tastes fabulously rich and creamy, but it's actually pretty low in fat, particularly if you use semi-skimmed milk.

MAKES **1 TALL GLASS**

1 large banana
3 tablespoons raisins, roughly chopped
2 tablespoons rum
150ml milk

1. Peel and slice the banana, pack into a freezerproof container and freeze for about 1½ hours until frozen.
2. Meanwhile, put the raisins in a small bowl, pour over the rum and leave to soak.
3. Put the frozen banana, reserving 1 slice to decorate, soaked raisins and rum, and milk in a food processor or blender and blend until thick and smooth. Pour the smoothie into a tall glass, decorate with a slice of banana and serve immediately.

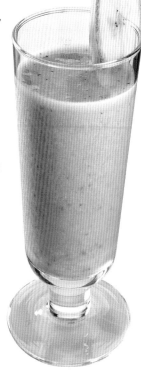

THINK PINK

RASPBERRY & ORANGE

Sweet, sharp, zesty and zingy, this fabulously slushy bright pink ice is similar to an Italian granita. The crystals of flavour melt on your tongue, releasing the delicious fresh fruit flavours around the mouth as you suck them off a spoon.

MAKES 4 GLASSES

500g raspberries
500ml orange juice
1–2 tablespoons icing sugar

1. Put the raspberries in a food processor or blender and blend to a purée. Place a sieve over a bowl and press the raspberry purée through the sieve to remove the pips. Stir in the orange juice and sugar to taste.

2. Pour the mixture into a freezerproof container and freeze for about 1 hour until the mixture freezes around the edges of the container.

3. Break up the mixture with a fork, then return to the freezer for a further 2 hours, breaking up the ice with a fork every 30 minutes until the mixture is slushy. Spoon into 4 glasses and serve immediately.

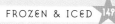

AROMATIC GRAPEFRUIT GRANITA

SUGAR, PINK GRAPEFRUIT & BASIL

Sweet, icy granitas are the perfect refresher in summer when it's blazing hot outside. Grapefruit is particularly good, with its sharp-sweet flavour that almost makes the taste buds tingle.

MAKES **4 GLASSES**

115g caster sugar
200ml water
3 pink grapefruit, halved
Fresh basil leaves, to garnish

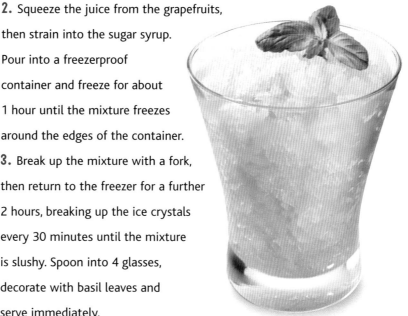

1. Put the sugar and water in a small pan and warm gently, stirring, until the sugar has dissolved. Bring to the boil, remove from the heat and leave to cool. Pour into a jug and chill.

2. Squeeze the juice from the grapefruits, then strain into the sugar syrup. Pour into a freezerproof container and freeze for about 1 hour until the mixture freezes around the edges of the container.

3. Break up the mixture with a fork, then return to the freezer for a further 2 hours, breaking up the ice crystals every 30 minutes until the mixture is slushy. Spoon into 4 glasses, decorate with basil leaves and serve immediately.

ISLAND YOGURT FROSTEE

PERSIMMON, BANANA, MANGO, PINEAPPLE & YOGURT

Thick, sweet and frosty like an old-fashioned milkshake, this yummy semi-frozen tropical smoothie is just the thing when you need an icy treat. Serve it for dessert with a teaspoon or as a refresher on a hot afternoon instead of ice cream.

MAKES **4 GLASSES**

2 persimmons, peeled
2 bananas, peeled
2 mangoes, pitted and peeled
4cm slice of pineapple, peeled
  and cored (about 75g)
240ml Greek yogurt

1. Roughly chop the fruit, put in a food processor or blender and blend until smooth.

2. Stir in the Greek yogurt, then pour the mixture into a freezerproof container and freeze for about 1 hour until the mixture freezes around the edges of the container.

3. Break up the mixture with a fork and freeze for a further 1–2 hours, mashing with a fork every 30 minutes until the mixture is thick and slushy. Spoon into 4 glasses and serve immediately.

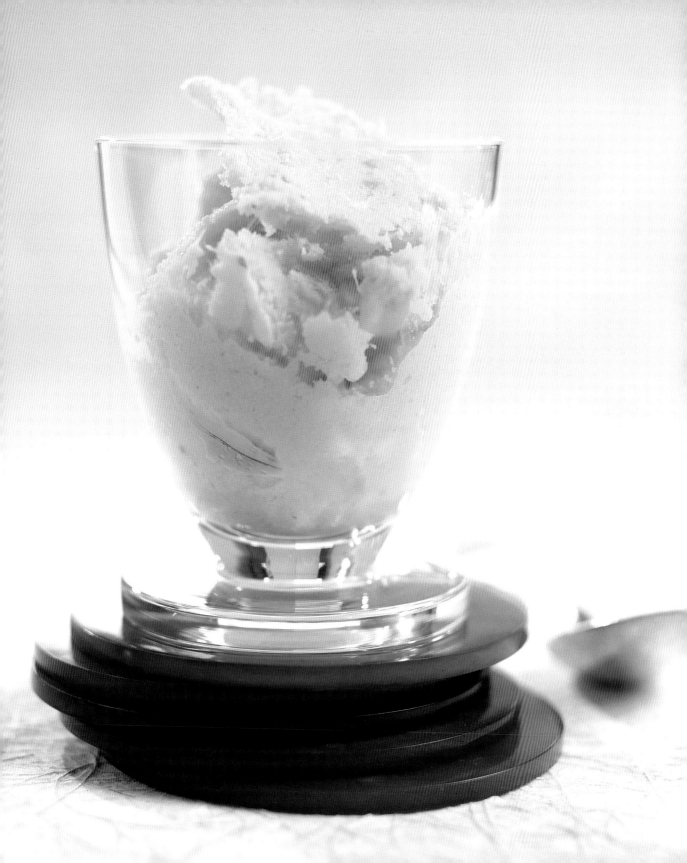

FRUITY ROSEMARY SEMIFREDDO

ROSEMARY, CRÈME FRAÎCHE & NECTARINE

The subtle hint of rosemary that shines through in this fruity, creamy semi-frozen smoothie highlights and accentuates the intense sweet-sharp flavour of nectarine perfectly. If you want to go for a super-healthy version, you can use plain yogurt instead of the crème fraîche if you prefer.

MAKES 4 GLASSES

4 sprigs of fresh rosemary, plus extra to decorate
125ml water
$1\frac{1}{2}$ tablespoons sugar
4 large, ripe nectarines, pitted
6 tablespoons crème fraîche

1. Put the rosemary in a small pan with the water and sugar and bring to the boil. Reduce the heat and simmer for 1 minute. Remove from the heat and leave to infuse for 20 minutes. Remove the rosemary and leave to cool completely.

2. Put the nectarines in a food processor or blender and strain the cooled rosemary syrup on top. Add the crème fraîche and blend until smooth.

3. Pour the mixture into a freezerproof container. Cover and freeze for about 1 hour until the mixture freezes around the edges of the container.

4. Break up the mixture with a fork, mashing it into the liquid and freeze for a further 2 hours, mashing with a fork every 30 minutes until the mixture is thick but still soft. Spoon into 4 glasses, decorate with a sprig of fresh rosemary and serve immediately.

VIRGIN PIÑA COLADA

PINEAPPLE, LIME & COCONUT

You can use fresh or canned pineapple to make this rich and creamy semi-frozen slush – making it the perfect choice when you're in the mood for an instant storecupboard frostee.

MAKES 4 GLASSES

600g prepared pineapple chunks
  or slices
240ml coconut milk
Juice of ½ lime
Lime rind or coconut shavings,
  to decorate

1. Put the pineapple in a food processor or blender and blend to a smooth purée. Press the purée through a sieve to remove the rough fibres.

2. Stir the coconut milk into the sieved purée and add lime juice to taste.

3. Pour the mixture into a freezerproof container and freeze for about 1 hour until the mixture freezes around the edges of the container.

4. Break up the mixture with a fork, mashing it into the liquid and freeze for a further 2 hours, mashing with a fork every 30 minutes until the mixture is thick but still soft. Spoon into 4 glasses, decorate with coconut shavings or rind and serve immediately.

TROPICAL SORBET BLEND

PASSION FRUIT, ORANGE & MANGO

This sweet, intensely flavoured sorbet-smoothie is the ideal refresher when it's blazing hot outside and you feel as though you're wilting in the heat. The tongue-tingling flavours and bite of sugary sharpness are sure to perk you up and revitalize you.

MAKES 1 GLASS

4 passion fruits
2 oranges, halved
2 scoops of mango sorbet

1. Halve the passion fruit and scoop the seeds and pulp into a sieve placed over a bowl. Press the seeds with the back of a spoon to extract all the juice and then discard the seeds.

2. Squeeze the juice from the oranges and pour into a food processor or blender with the passion fruit juice.

3. Add 1 scoop of mango sorbet and blend briefly to combine. Pour into a glass, add the second scoop of sorbet and serve immediately.

SCENTED GRAPE SLUSH

GRAPE

Because grapes are naturally so sweet, you don't need to add any extra sugar to this granita-style slush. Choose well-flavoured grapes with a scented flavour such as muscat grapes for the best flavour and serve as an icy refresher on a hot summer's day.

MAKES **2 GLASSES**

600g grapes

1. Put the grapes in a food processor or blender and blend until mushy. Tip into a sieve over a bowl, squeeze out all the juice using the back of a spoon and discard the grape skins.

2. Pour the mixture into a freezerproof container. Cover and freeze for about 30 minutes until the mixture freezes around the edges of the container.

3. Break up the mixture with a fork, mashing it into the liquid and freeze for a further 2 hours, breaking up the ice with a fork every 30 minutes until the mixture is thick and slushy. Spoon into 2 glasses and serve immediately.

WATERMELON & STEM GINGER ICE

WATERMELON, STEM GINGER & LIME

Sharp, sweet and with the peppery bite of ginger, this slushy, granita-style ice offers the ultimate in cooling refreshers. It's great in summer when watermelons are in season and at their gorgeous, ruby-coloured best.

MAKES 4 GLASSES

1kg watermelon
2 balls of stem ginger, plus 2
   tablespoons syrup from the jar
Juice of 1½ limes
A few strips of lime rind,
   to decorate

1. Remove the seeds from the watermelon, then cut away the skin. Put the flesh in a food processor or blender with the ginger and syrup and blend until smooth.

2. Stir in the lime juice to taste and then pour the mixture into a freezerproof container. Freeze for about 1 hour until the mixture freezes around the edges of the container.

3. Break up the mixture with a fork, then return to the freezer for a further 2 hours, breaking up with a fork every 30 minutes until the mixture is slushy. Spoon into 4 glasses, decorate with lime rind and serve immediately.

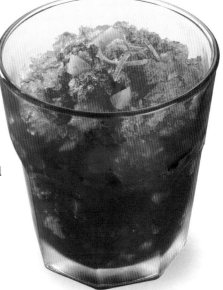

CREAMY, FROTHY ICED LATTE

MILK, CREAM & ESPRESSO

Sweet, slushy and packing that inimitable caffeine punch, this is the iced coffee that's perfect served at any time of day – it'll wake you up first thing, perk you up mid-morning or mid-afternoon and makes the ideal dessert-coffee combo when you haven't got time for a proper pud.

MAKES **1 TALL GLASS**

1 glass crushed ice
125ml milk
2 tablespoons double cream
3 tablespoons freshly brewed
  espresso
1 tablespoon caster sugar

1. Put the ice in a food processor or blender and pour over the milk, cream, espresso and sugar. Blend until frothy and slushy.

2. Pour into a tall glass and serve immediately.

CINNAMON FROSTY SHAKE

APPLE, CINNAMON & VANILLA ICE CREAM

Fragrant cinnamon creates a sensationally moreish flavouring in this sweet, frothy shake. Choose sharp, well-flavoured apples such as Braeburns or Coxes for juicing so they really offset the sweetness of the ice cream and balance the aromatic spice of the cinnamon.

MAKES 1 GLASS

4 dessert apples
$\frac{1}{4}$ teaspoon ground cinnamon
Handful of crushed ice
2 large scoops of vanilla ice cream
Apple slices or fresh blackberries,
   to decorate

1. Cut the apples into wedges then press through a juicer.

2. Pour the juice into a food processor or blender and add the cinnamon, crushed ice and one scoop of ice cream. Blend until frothy.

3. Pour into a glass, add the second scoop of ice cream and decorate with apple slices or blackberries. Serve immediately.

TUTTI FRUTTI SHAKE

PINEAPPLE, VANILLA ICE CREAM & GLACÉ CHERRY

Inspired by the classic Italian ice cream, whose name means 'all the fruits', this pretty cherry-flecked shake is perfect for summer. With its sweet, tropical taste of pineapple and the pretty flecks of cherry colouring the shake, it will appeal to everyone – both young and old.

MAKES 1 GLASS

230g pineapple chunks
60ml pineapple juice
2 scoops of vanilla ice cream
5 multicoloured glacé cherries, roughly chopped, plus extra to decorate

1. Put the pineapple chunks, juice and ice cream in a food processor or blender and blend until smooth.
2. Add the cherries and blitz briefly until chopped and the shake is flecked with pieces of cherry. Pour into a glass, decorate with glacé cherries threaded onto a cocktail stick and serve immediately.

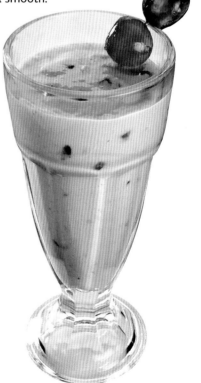

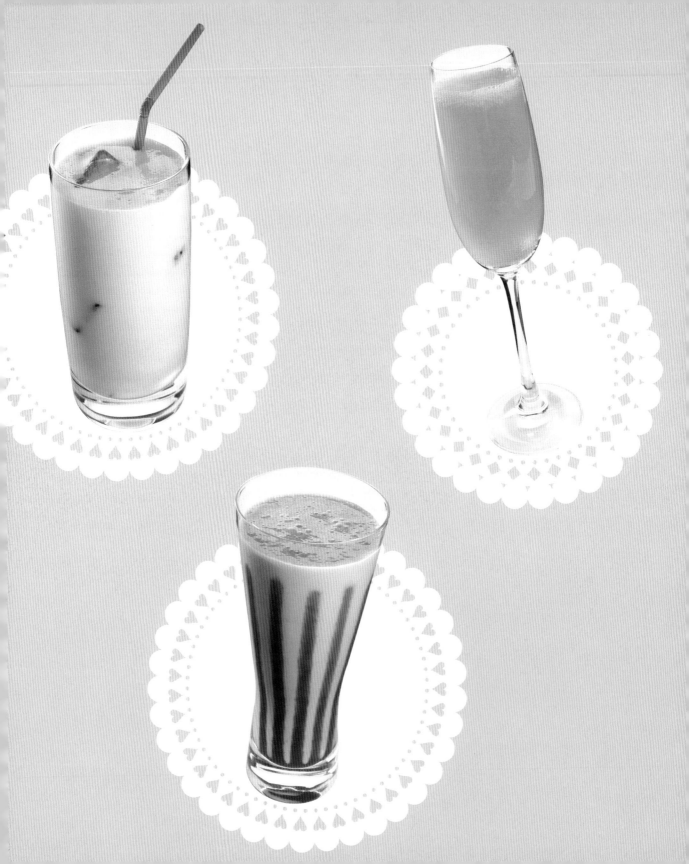

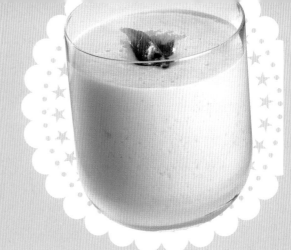

NAUGHTY BUT NICE

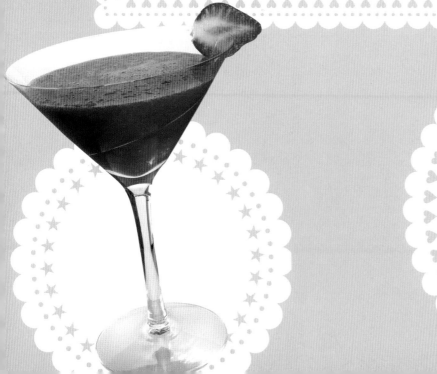

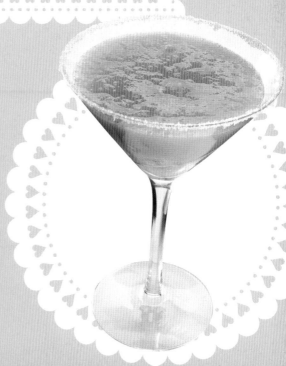

SEA BREEZE

GRAPEFRUIT, CRANBERRY & VODKA

Nothing beats a freshly juiced Sea Breeze. Fresh, fruity and with that deliciously sharp-sour kick of grapefruit, cranberry and vodka, it makes the perfect tipple to serve as an aperitif or cocktail to sip all night long.

MAKES 1 TALL GLASS

½ pink or ruby grapefruit
Crushed ice or ice cubes
3 tablespoons vodka
75ml cranberry juice
Lime wedges, to serve

1. Squeeze the juice from the grapefruit.

2. Fill a tall glass with ice and pour over the vodka.

3. Next, pour over the grapefruit juice and cranberry juice and finish with a lime wedge. Jiggle with a stirrer and serve immediately.

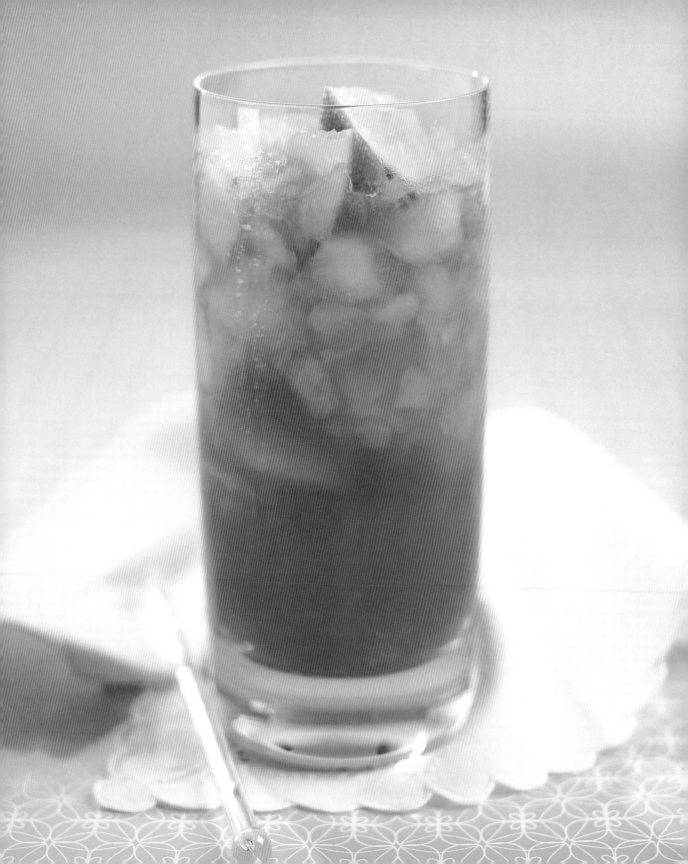

FRUITY STRAWBERRY DAIQUIRI

STRAWBERRY, LIME & RUM

Sweet, sharp and fruity, daiquiris are the ultimate Cuban cocktail – perfect for sipping on the beach, but even better for serving up at a party. Banana daiquiris are another classic flavouring, so try making a variation using half a banana in place of the strawberries if you like.

MAKES 1 GLASS

4 large strawberries, hulled (about 75g), plus extra to decorate
3 tablespoons white rum
Juice of 1 lime
1 tablespoon icing sugar
125ml crushed ice

1. Put the strawberries, rum, lime juice, sugar and ice in a food processor or blender and blend until smooth.

2. Pour into a glass and serve immediately. Decorate with a slice of strawberry.

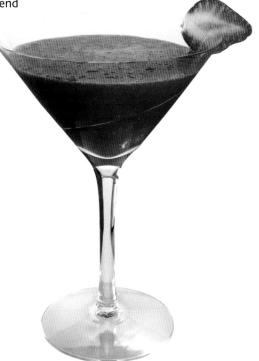

BOOZY FESTIVE SMOOTHIE

PRUNE, FIG, YOGURT, MILK, CRÈME FRAÎCHE, BRANDY & HONEY

This lusciously indulgent thick and creamy smoothie tastes like an extra
creamy Christmas pudding in a glass. Look out for festive drink stirrers
or long-handled spoons around Christmas-time to pop in your glass.

MAKES **1 GLASS**

4 ready-to-eat dried prunes, pitted
2 ready-to-eat dried figs
75ml plain yogurt
150ml milk
2 tablespoons crème fraîche
2 tablespoons brandy
1 teaspoon clear honey

1. Put the prunes, figs, yogurt, milk, crème fraîche, brandy and honey in
a food processor or blender and blend until smooth, creamy and frothy.

2. Pour into a glass and serve immediately.

SPARKLING PARTY PUNCH

APPLE, STRAWBERRY, COINTREAU & WINE

When you're throwing a party, it's great to mix up a large jug of punch so that you can serve guests quickly and easily. This fresh and fruity concoction is just perfect for summer when strawberries are in season. If you like, you can also mix up the drinks in glasses. Simply divide the strawberry-Cointreau mix between six champagne flutes and top up with sparkling wine individually.

MAKES 6 GLASSES

3 apples or 175ml apple juice
250g strawberries
75ml Cointreau
1 bottle chilled sparkling wine

1. If using whole apples, cut into wedges and press through a juicer.
2. Pour the apple juice into a food processor or blender with the strawberries and blend until smooth.
3. Pour the fruit purée into a large bowl or jug and stir in the Cointreau. Add the sparkling wine and stir to combine. Pour into 6 glasses and serve.

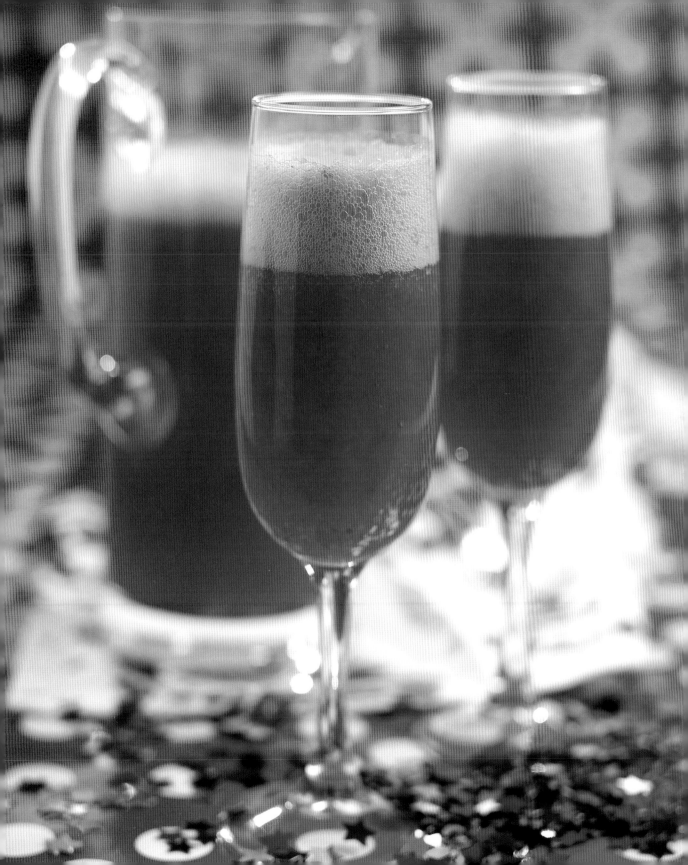

PASSION FRUIT MIMOSA

PASSION FRUIT, ORANGE & CHAMPAGNE

The classic Mimosa is made with orange juice and
champagne, but this fragrant version is made with the
addition of passion fruit, which adds a tantalizing tang.
If you're making it for a party, you can juice the fruit
beforehand and store in the fridge so it's ready to serve
when your guests arrive.

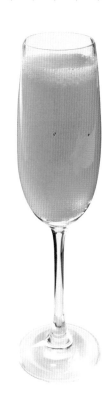

MAKES 6 GLASSES

6 passion fruit
6 oranges, halved
1 bottle chilled champagne

1. Halve the passion fruits, scoop the flesh into a sieve and then press
through to extract the pulp.
2. Squeeze the juice from the oranges and add to the passion fruit pulp.
Stir together well.
3. Divide the fruit juice between 6 champagne flutes or saucers, top up
with champagne and serve immediately.

PINEAPPLE & RUM SMOOTHIE

PINEAPPLE, YOGURT & RUM

This tropical cocktail blend adds a boozy twist to an otherwise super-healthy smoothie. If you want to go for the healthy option, you can leave out the rum as it tastes just as good without. Use canned or fresh pineapple – either will taste great.

MAKES **1 GLASS**

150g prepared pineapple slices or
   chunks
80ml plain yogurt
4 tablespoons pineapple juice
1$\frac{1}{2}$ tablespoons white rum

1. Put the pineapple, yogurt and pineapple juice in a food processor or blender and blend until smooth.

2. Strain the mixture through a sieve to remove any rough pulp, using the back of a spoon to ease the mixture through.

3. Pour the smoothie into a glass, stir in the rum and serve immediately.

CHERRY TRIFLE SMOOTHIE

CHERRY, MILK, CUSTARD & CREAM

Thick, rich and tangily indulgent, this smoothie is one to linger over with a long-handled spoon so you can get right to the bottom of the glass, scraping up every last delicious drop.

MAKES 1 GLASS

200g black cherries, plus extra
   to decorate
1 tablespoon milk
75ml chilled fresh custard
2 tablespoons double cream
2 sponge fingers

1. Remove the stalks and stones from the cherries. If you don't have a cherry-pitter, cut arond the crease of each cherry, gently prize the two halves and pull out the stone.

2. Put the cherries in a food processor or blender and blend to a smooth purée.

3. In a separate jug, stir the milk into the custard until smooth and creamy and of pouring consistency.

4. In a bowl, whip the cream until it holds in soft peaks.

5. Spoon layers of the custard mixture and cherry purée into a glass, top with a generous dollop of whipped cream and decorate with a few fresh cherries.

6. Stick a couple of sponge fingers on top and serve with a long-handled spoon.

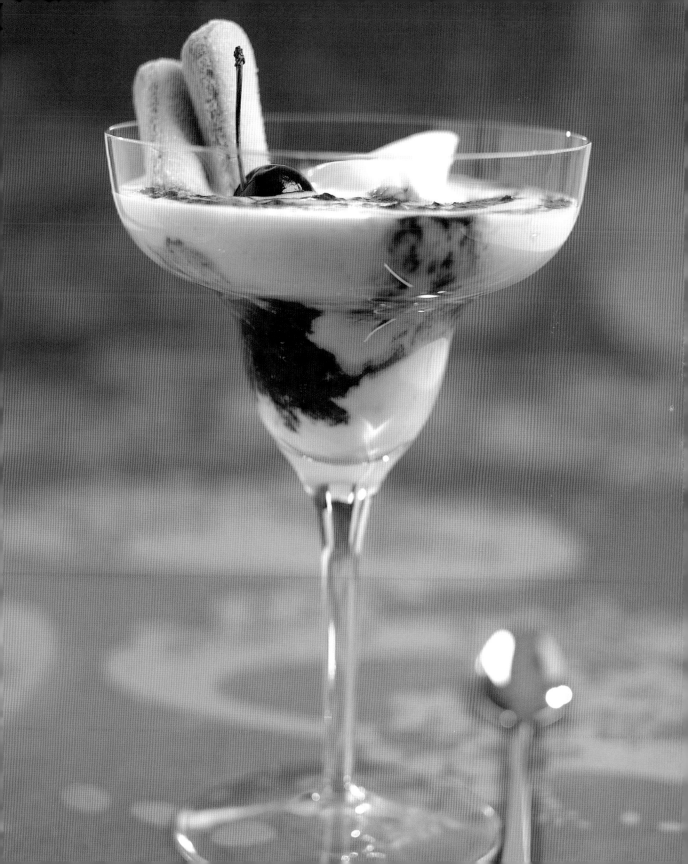

PEACH MELBA SMOOTHIE

PEACH, RASPBERRY, CUSTARD & MILK

This rich, fruity vanilla smoothie was inspired by the classic dessert Peach Melba, made with fresh peaches, raspberry purée and vanilla ice cream. This version offers a surprise in every mouthful with the sweet velvety taste of vanilla custard, the sharpness of raspberries and the luxurious scented flavour of peaches or mango – depending on which you choose.

MAKES 1 GLASS

1 large peach, pitted or ½ small
  mango, pitted and peeled
100g raspberries, plus extra
  to decorate
75ml vanilla custard
2 tablespoons milk

1. Put the peach or mango flesh in a food processor or blender and blend until smooth. Transfer to a small bowl and set aside.

2. Rinse out the food processor or blender, blend the raspberries to make a purée and set aside.

3. Stir the custard and milk together until smooth and of pouring consistency, then set aside.

4. Spoon alternate layers of peach or mango purée, raspberry purée and custard into a glass, decorate with fresh raspberries and serve immediately.

ZING-A-LING

YOGURT, MILK, GINGER & MAPLE SYRUP

This sweet, zingy, peppery smoothie has a wonderfully
indulgent, tantalizing flavour. Choose a really mild-tasting
yogurt such as live 'bio' yogurt so the taste of maple and
ginger really shines through. You can store any leftover
praline in an airtight container for later use.

MAKES 1 GLASS

125ml plain yogurt
100ml milk
$1\frac{1}{2}$ balls stem of ginger in syrup
1 tablespoon maple syrup

FOR THE PRALINE
30g pecan nuts, roughly chopped
60g caster sugar

1. First make the praline decoration. Line a baking sheet with greaseproof
paper and spread over the nuts so slightly spaced. Put the sugar in a dry
pan and heat gently for about 5 minutes or until the syrup is pale golden.
Pour over the nuts on the lined baking sheet. Leave to harden for
about 20 minutes, then break into shards.

2. Put the yogurt, milk, ginger
and syrup in a food processor
or blender and blend for about
1 minute until thoroughly blended
and smooth.

3. Pour into a glass and decorate
with shards of praline to serve.

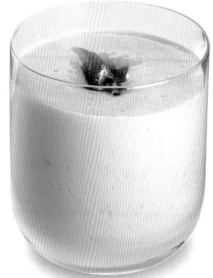

APRICOT & AMARETTI SMOOTHIE

APRICOT, YOGURT, MILK & AMARETTI

Rich, smooth and creamy, with the unmistakably sweet, scented flavour of almonds combined with the subtle sharpness of apricots, this indulgent smoothie makes a great alternative to dessert. But don't feel you have to save it for dessert – it really is wonderful any time.

MAKES 1 TALL GLASS

4 ready-to-eat dried apricots
3 tablespoons Greek yogurt
100ml milk
5 small amaretti (about 15g),
   plus extra to decorate
Crushed ice or ice cubes,
   to serve

1. Put the apricots, yogurt, milk and amaretti in a food processor or blender and blend until really smooth and frothy.
2. Place the ice in a tall glass, then pour in the smoothie, decorate with crushed amaretti and serve immediately.

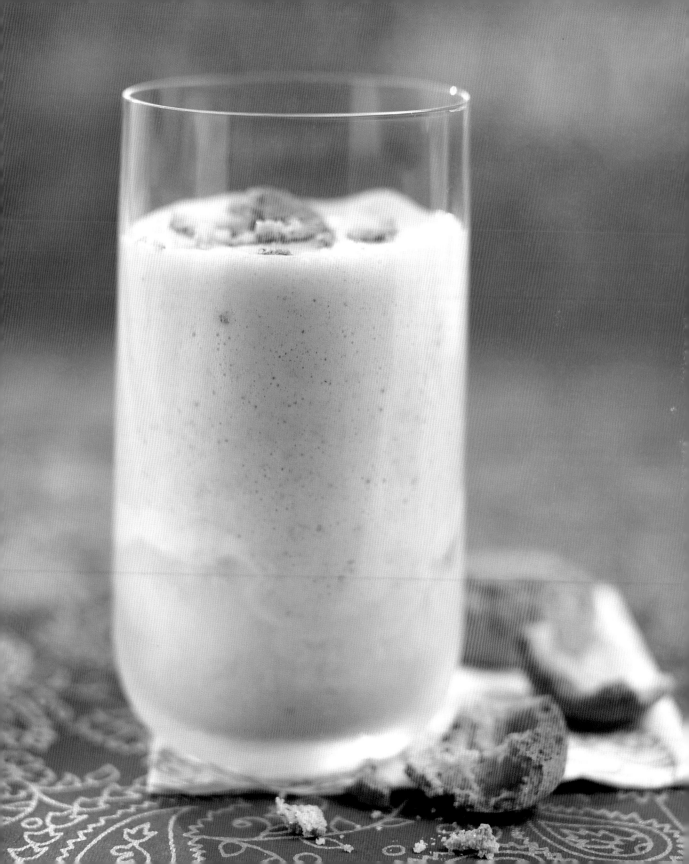

ROSEWATER DELIGHT

NECTARINE, ROSEWATER, MILK & HONEY

The scented flavour of rosewater gives this deliciously rich and creamy smoothie a real taste of the Middle East. For the best results, look out for juicy, well-flavoured nectarines.

MAKES 1 GLASS

1 large, ripe nectarine, pitted and
  roughly chopped
$1\frac{1}{2}$ teaspoons rosewater
100ml milk
75ml Greek yogurt
$\frac{1}{2}$ teaspoon clear honey
Ice cubes, to serve
Pale pink rose petals, to decorate

1. Put the nectarine, rosewater, milk, yogurt and honey in a food processor or blender and blend until smooth, creamy and frothy.

2. Pour into a glass, add a few ice cubes and decorate with pale pink rose petals to serve.

THICK & CREAMY RHUBARB SMOOTHIE

RHUBARB, YOGURT & MILK

This sharp, sweet, silky smoothie is simply delicious. Make it with early-season forced rhubarb to get a really delicate, perfectly pretty-pink colour. If you prefer your smoothie on the sweet side, add a little more sugar to taste, or if you prefer it sharp, leave it just as it is with that unmistakable rhubarb bite.

MAKES 1 GLASS

1 stick of rhurbarb (about 115g), chopped
1 tablespoon caster sugar
1 tablespoon water
2 tablespoons Greek yogurt
80ml milk
Ice cubes, to serve

1. Put the rhubarb, sugar and water in a pan, cover with a lid and heat gently, shaking occasionally until the water simmers. Cook for about 5 minutes until tender, remove from the heat and leave to cool.

2. Put the cooled rhubarb, yogurt and milk in a food processor or blender and blend until smooth and frothy. Check for sweetness and add a little more sugar if necessary and whizz again to combine.

3. Add a few ice cubes to a glass, then pour in the smoothie and serve immediately.

CHOCALICIOUS KAHLUA BROWNIE MILKSHAKE

CHOCOLATE BROWNIE, MILK, YOGURT & KAHLUA

Unbelievably simple to make but tasting like a million dollars, this sweet, sticky and slightly alchoholic shake is just the thing when you need a sugary pick-me-up. If you want to make a child-friendly version just miss out the kahlua. They'll love the non-alcoholic version just as much.

MAKES 1 TALL GLASS

1 chocolate brownie (about 50g)
175ml milk
1 tablespoon Greek yogurt
1 tablespoon Kahlua

1. Break the brownie into chunks and put in a food processor or blender with the milk, yogurt and Kahlua. Blend until really smooth and frothy.

2. Pour into a tall glass and serve immediately with a long straw.

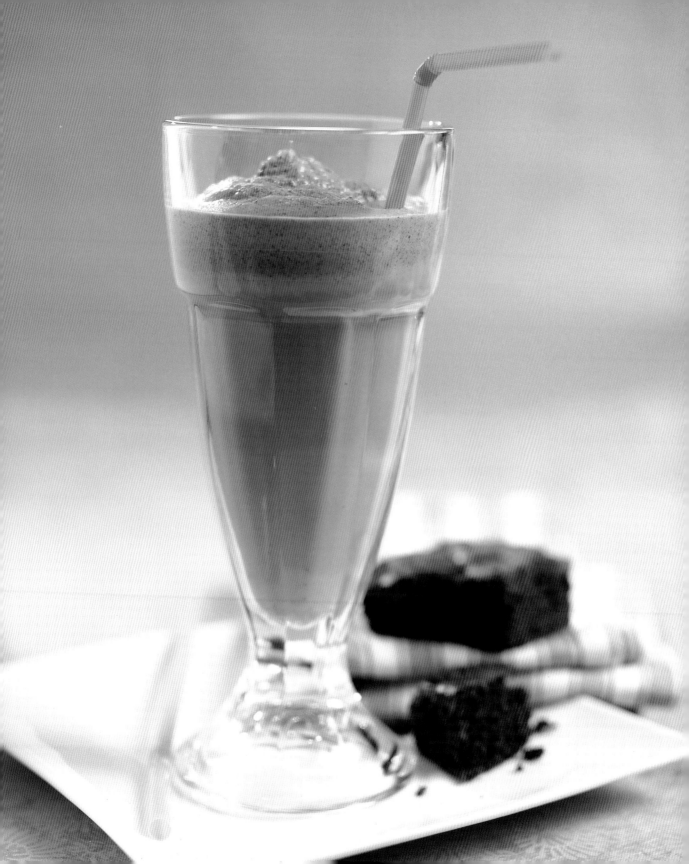

BANOFFEE SMOOTHIE

BANANA, MILK, YOGURT, CREAM & TOFFEE

Rich, creamy and utterly irresistible, you'll find this sweet and sticky treat almost velvety on the lips when you sip it. Wickedly luxurious, indulge yourself when you're down in the dumps – or on top of the world!

MAKES 1 TALL GLASS

1 banana
125ml milk
4 tablespoons plain yogurt
2 tablespoons double cream
2 tablespoons dulce de leche, plus
   extra to serve

1. Peel the banana and cut into chunks, then put in a food processor or blender with the milk, yogurt, cream and dulce de leche. Blend until smooth and frothy.
2. Drizzle lines of dulce de leche inside a tall glass, then pour in the smoothie and serve.

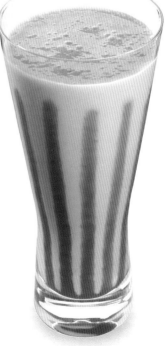

MARZIPAN MADNESS

ORANGE, MARZIPAN & YOGURT

This rich, indulgent smoothie is a fabulous combination of smooth, creamy, sharp and sweet with the intense flavour of freshly juiced oranges shining through and the subtle underlying scent of almonds flirting just underneath.

MAKES 1 GLASS

2 oranges, halved
2 tablespoons finely grated marzipan
    (about 20g)
4 tablespoons plain yogurt
Ice cubes, to serve (optional)

1. Squeeze the juice from the oranges and pour into a food processor or blender, add the marzipan and yogurt and blend until really smooth and frothy.

2. Pour into a glass, add a few ice cubes, if liked, and serve immediately.

VANILLA & NOUGAT SMOOTHIE

NOUGAT, YOGURT AND MILK

This intensely sweet, creamy smoothie is at its best served ice cold and sipped slowly. Make it in a jug blender with a lid rather than with a hand-held wand blender, because the hard nougat is liable to make the mixture spit and splash as you blend it.

MAKES 1 GLASS

40g nougat, chopped
4 tablespoons thick and creamy
   vanilla yogurt
150ml milk
Ice cubes, to serve

1. Put the nougat, yogurt and milk in a food processor or blender and blend for about 1 minute until very smooth and creamy.

2. Half fill a glass with ice, then pour over the smoothie and serve immediately.

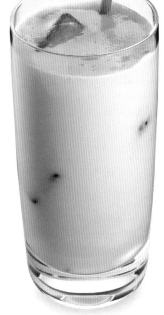

ETON MESS IN A GLASS

STRAWBERRY, YOGURT, CREAM & MERINGUE

Inspired by the classic dessert, Eton Mess, this gloriously indulgent smoothie really is heaven in a glass. Flecked with tiny crumbs of sweet meringue, this rich, creamy, pink smoothie is the ultimate in feel-good pick-me-ups.

MAKES 1 GLASS

120g strawberries, hulled
100ml plain yogurt
3 tablespoons double cream
2 meringue nests, broken into pieces

1. Reserve one strawberry to decorate. Cut it into slices and set aside.

2. Put the rest of the strawberries in a food processor or blender with the yogurt and double cream and blend until smooth and frothy.

3. Add about three-quarters of the meringue, blitz for a second or two until just combined and then pour into a glass.

4. Sprinkle over the remaining pieces of meringue, decorate with the slices of strawberry and serve immediately.

LEMON MERINGUE CREAM

YOGURT, CRÈME FRAÎCHE, MILK, LEMON & MERINGUE

For a really rich, lemony flavour, use a good-quality lemon curd for this fabulously indulgent smoothie. It looks simply stunning served pure and virginal with the creamy smoothie topped with snow-white meringue, but it's lovely with a few blueberries sprinkled on top too.

MAKES 1 GLASS

5 tablespoons plain yogurt
3 tablespoons crème fraîche
90ml milk
3 tablespoons good-quality
   lemon curd
1 meringue nest, crumbled
Small handful of fresh blueberries,
   to decorate (optional)

1. Put the yogurt, crème fraîche, milk and lemon curd in a food processor or blender and blend until smooth and creamy. Check the flavour and add a little more lemon curd, if necessary.

2. Pour the smoothie into a glass and sprinkle the meringue on top. Scatter a few blueberries on top, if liked, and serve immediately.

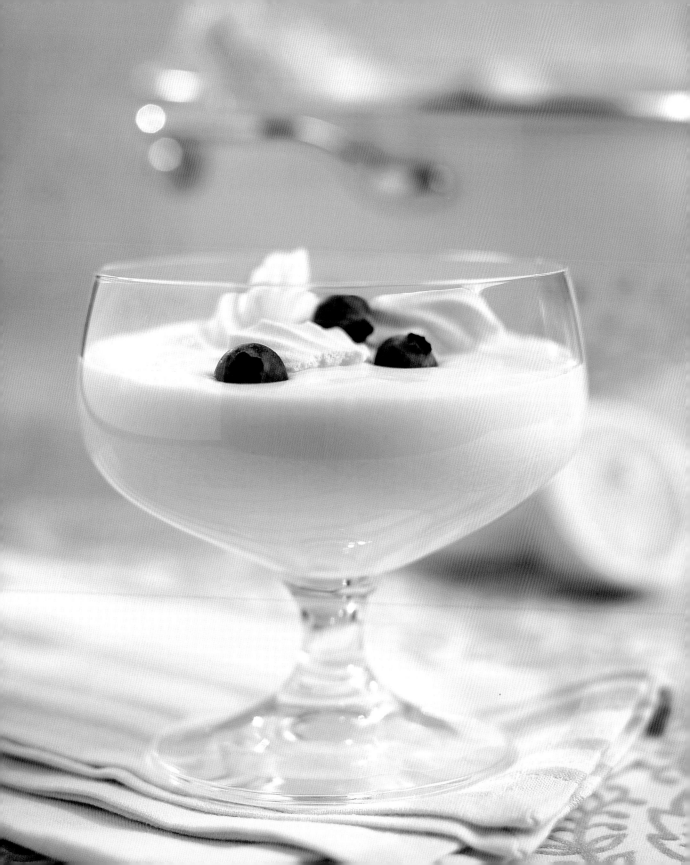

MANGO MARGARITA

MANGO, TEQUILA, GRAND MARNIER & LIME

This twist on the classic Mexican drink turns a cheeky cocktail into a
luxurious smoothie, and a velvety smoothie into a wickedly indulgent treat!
Use really ripe, sweet, scented mangoes for the best results.

MAKES 4 GLASSES

Juice of 2 limes
Salt, to serve
2 mangoes
125ml tequila
60ml Grand Marnier
240ml crushed ice

1. First, rub a little lime juice around the rim of 4 margarita glasses, then dip the rims in salt and set aside.

2. Using a small, sharp knife, remove the peel from the mango, then slice the flesh away from the stone.

3. Put the mangoes, tequila, Grand Marnier and lime juice in a food processor or blender and blend until smooth.

4. Add the ice and blend again until slushy. Pour into the prepared margarita glasses and serve immediately.

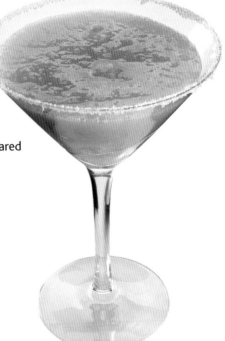

CAIPIRINHA

LIME, SUGAR & CACHAÇA

This fabulous zingy, zesty, energizing tipple made with fresh lime juice is the national cocktail of Brazil and is sure to get any party going with true South American style. Cachaça is made from distilled sugar cane juice, but if you can't get hold of this marvellous Brazilian liquor you can use rum instead. It will give a slightly different flavour — but it won't affect your party in the slightest!

MAKES 1 GLASS

1 lime, quartered
2 teaspoons demerara sugar
Ice (crushed or whole cubes)
3 tablespoons cachaça

1. Put the lime quarters in a sturdy tumbler and gently crush them with the end of a rolling pin to release the juice.

2. Sprinkle over the sugar and muddle until the sugar has dissolved.

3. Fill the glass with ice, then pour over the cachaça and stir to combine. Serve immediately.

INDEX

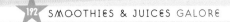

PHOTOGRAPHY CREDITS

IAN GARLICK

PAGES: 29, 35, 39, 45, 49, 53, 57, 61, 65, 69, 75, 79, 83, 87, 93, 97, 101, 103, 105, 108, 112, 117, 121, 125, 129, 133, 137, 141, 145, 151, 163, 167, 171, 175, 179, 183,

SIMON PASK

PAGES: 37, 42, 63, 76, 94, 114, 115, 122, 126, 131, 139, 142, 147, 149, 153, 155, 156, 159, 164, 169, 173, 180, 184